Jolanta Siller-Matula

**Thrombin as a multifunctional enzyme**

Jolanta Siller-Matula

# Thrombin as a multifunctional enzyme
## Establishing experimental models to study thrombin effects

Südwestdeutscher Verlag für Hochschulschriften

**Impressum/Imprint (nur für Deutschland/only for Germany)**
Bibliografische Information der Deutschen Nationalbibliothek: Die Deutsche Nationalbibliothek verzeichnet diese Publikation in der Deutschen Nationalbibliografie; detaillierte bibliografische Daten sind im Internet über http://dnb.d-nb.de abrufbar.
Alle in diesem Buch genannten Marken und Produktnamen unterliegen warenzeichen-, marken- oder patentrechtlichem Schutz bzw. sind Warenzeichen oder eingetragene Warenzeichen der jeweiligen Inhaber. Die Wiedergabe von Marken, Produktnamen, Gebrauchsnamen, Handelsnamen, Warenbezeichnungen u.s.w. in diesem Werk berechtigt auch ohne besondere Kennzeichnung nicht zu der Annahme, dass solche Namen im Sinne der Warenzeichen- und Markenschutzgesetzgebung als frei zu betrachten wären und daher von jedermann benutzt werden dürften.

Verlag: Südwestdeutscher Verlag für Hochschulschriften GmbH & Co. KG
Dudweiler Landstr. 99, 66123 Saarbrücken, Deutschland
Telefon +49 681 37 20 271-1, Telefax +49 681 37 20 271-0
Email: info@svh-verlag.de

Approved by: Medizinische Universität Wien, Dissertation, 2011

Herstellung in Deutschland:
Schaltungsdienst Lange o.H.G., Berlin
Books on Demand GmbH, Norderstedt
Reha GmbH, Saarbrücken
Amazon Distribution GmbH, Leipzig
**ISBN: 978-3-8381-2908-2**

**Imprint (only for USA, GB)**
Bibliographic information published by the Deutsche Nationalbibliothek: The Deutsche Nationalbibliothek lists this publication in the Deutsche Nationalbibliografie; detailed bibliographic data are available in the Internet at http://dnb.d-nb.de.
Any brand names and product names mentioned in this book are subject to trademark, brand or patent protection and are trademarks or registered trademarks of their respective holders. The use of brand names, product names, common names, trade names, product descriptions etc. even without a particular marking in this works is in no way to be construed to mean that such names may be regarded as unrestricted in respect of trademark and brand protection legislation and could thus be used by anyone.

Publisher: Südwestdeutscher Verlag für Hochschulschriften GmbH & Co. KG
Dudweiler Landstr. 99, 66123 Saarbrücken, Germany
Phone +49 681 37 20 271-1, Fax +49 681 37 20 271-0
Email: info@svh-verlag.de

Printed in the U.S.A.
Printed in the U.K. by (see last page)
**ISBN: 978-3-8381-2908-2**

Copyright © 2011 by the author and Südwestdeutscher Verlag für Hochschulschriften GmbH & Co. KG and licensors
All rights reserved. Saarbrücken 2011

## ACKNOWLEDGEMENT

I am heartily thankful to my family for their love, encouragement and help in reaching my academic goals. Especially, I would like to show my gratitude to my parents who supported me in all my pursuits. And most of all I want to thank my loving husband Christian, whose faithful support during this Ph.D. is so appreciated.

Thank you

# TABLE OF CONTENTS

- ABSTRACT ................................................................................. 6
- 1. INTRODUCTION ...................................................................... 7
  - 1.1. Identification of thrombin ................................................. 7
  - 1.2 Evolution of thrombin ....................................................... 7
  - 1.3 Biosynthesis of prothrombin ............................................. 8
  - 1.4 Structure of thrombin ....................................................... 8
  - 1.5. Thrombin and genetics ................................................... 9
  - 1.6. Functions of thrombin in coagulation ............................... 9
  - 1.7. Pleiotropic functions of thrombin ..................................... 10
    - 1.7.1. Protease activated receptors (PARs) ....................... 10
    - 1.7.2. Thrombin and platelets ............................................. 13
    - 1.7.3. Thrombin and cancer ............................................... 14
  - 1.8. Role of thrombin in disseminated intravascular coagulation (DIC) ......... 14
  - 1.9. Animal studies examining effects of thrombin in vivo ....... 15
  - 1.10. Use of thrombin as a therapeutic .................................. 20
  - 1.11. Use of thrombin inhibitors as a therapeutic ................... 21
- 2. RATIONALE AND STUDY AIMS ................................................ 22
- 3. METHODS ............................................................................... 23
  - 3.1. Design of studies ............................................................ 24
    - 3.1.1. STUDY I: Interspecies differences in coagulation profile with and without thrombin stimulation ............ 24
    - 3.1.2. STUDY II: A rat model of thrombin – induced consumption coagulopathy ................. 24
      - 3.1.2.1. Part I: dose escalation ...................................... 25
      - 3.1.2.2. Part II: dose verification ................................... 25
      - 3.1.2.3. Part III: lepirudin vs. placebo ........................... 25
    - 3.1.3. STUDY III: An ovine model of thrombin – induced consumption coagulopathy ................. 26
      - 3.1.3.1. Part I: dose escalation ...................................... 26
      - 3.1.3.2 Part II: dose verification .................................... 27
  - 3.2. Modified Rotation Thromboelastometry Analyzer (ROTEM) ........ 27
  - 3.3. Endogenous thrombin potential (ETP) ............................. 27
  - 3.4. Platelet Function Analyzer (PFA-100) .............................. 28

*Table of contents*

| | |
|---|---|
| 3.5. Impedance Aggregometry | 28 |
| 3.6. Von Willebrand Factor-Ristocetin Cofactor Activity (vWF:RICO) | 28 |
| 3.7. Two-dimensional electrophoresis (2-DE) | 29 |
| 3.8. Mass spectrometric analysis (MS) | 29 |
| 3.9. Other laboratory assays | 29 |
| 3.10. Measurement of the expression of MCP-1, IL6, TNF-alpha and IL-10 | 31 |
| 3.11. Tissue histology | 31 |
| 3.12. Data analysis | 31 |
|     3.12.1. Study I: Interspecies differences in coagulation profile with and without thrombin stimulation | 31 |
|     3.12.2. Study II: A rat model of thrombin – induced consumption coagulopathy | 31 |
|     3.12.3. Study III: An ovine model of thrombin – induced consumption coagulopathy | 32 |
| **4. RESULTS** | 33 |
| 4.1. Study I: Interspecies differences in coagulation profile with and without thrombin stimulation | 33 |
|     4.1.1. Interspecies differences measured by ROTEM | 33 |
|     4.1.2. Endogenous thrombin potential (ETP) | 35 |
|     4.1.3. Coagulation parameters at baseline | 36 |
| 4.2. Study II: A rat model of thrombin – induced consumption coagulopathy | 37 |
|     4.2.1. Dose escalation | 37 |
|         4.2.1.1. Laboratory parameters | 37 |
|         4.2.1.2. Inflammation parameters | 39 |
|         4.2.1.3. Association between thrombin dose, platelet count, fibrinogen level and IL-6 level | 39 |
|         4.2.1.4. Symptoms of DIC and survival | 40 |
|         4.2.1.5. Estimates of safety and tolerability | 42 |
|         4.2.1.6. Association between platelet count, fibrinogen level, bleeding events and survival | 42 |
|     4.2.2. Dose verification | 43 |
|     4.2.3. Lepirudin/Placebo | 43 |
| 4.3. Study III: An ovine model of thrombin – induced consumption coagulopathy | 46 |
|     4.3.1. Dose escalation | 46 |

*Table of contents*

      4.3.1.1. Coagulation parameters ............................................... 47

      4.3.1.2. Estimates of safety and tolerability ............................... 48

    4.3.2. Dose verification……..  ............................................................ 48

      4.3.2.1. Coagulation parameters ............................................... 48

      4.3.2.2. Proteomics and mass spectrometry analyses ................. 51

      4.3.2.3. Thromboelastometry ..................................................... 53

      4.3.2.4. Platelet Function ........................................................... 54

      4.3.2.5. Thrombin generation assay .......................................... 54

      4.3.2.6. Symptoms of DIC, Survival and Organ Pathology ............ 55

**5. DISCUSSION** ................................................................................................ 57

  5.1. Interspecies differences in coagulation profile ................................. 57

  5.2. Animal models of thrombin – induced consumption coagulopathy ......... 60

  5.3. Limitations ....................................................................................... 66

**6. CONCLUSIONS** ........................................................................................... 67

**7. REFERENCES** .............................................................................................. 68

  LIST OF ABBREVATIONS ...................................................................... 85

# ABSTRACT

**BACKGROUND AND AIMS:** Although several decades of research on thrombin functions have provided a framework for understanding the biology of thrombin, studies are still needed to further characterise the functions of thrombin in disease. The objectives of this thesis were to i) perform a cross-species comparison of clotting properties in order to characterise species, which mimic the coagulation profile in human most adequately and ii) establish rodent and non-rodent models of protracted intravenous thrombin infusion at steady state condition.

**METHODS:** In STUDY I (Interspecies differences in coagulation profile with and without thrombin stimulation) the *in vitro* effects of thrombin at doses of 0.0002-1 IU/ml were studied with thromboelastometry in blood from humans, rats, pigs, sheep and rabbits. In STUDY II (A rat model of thrombin – induced consumption coagulopathy) the *in vivo* effects of thrombin at doses 0.05-0.9IU/kg/min were studied in Sprague Dawley rats. In STUDY III (An ovine model of thrombin – induced consumption coagulopathy) the *in vivo* effects of thrombin at doses 0.0004-0.42IU/kg/min were studied in Austrian Mountain Sheep.

**RESULTS:** STUDY I: In humans and sheep, the clotting time was in the same range with or without thrombin stimulation and a 100-fold lower dose of thrombin was required to cause a shortening in the clotting time as compared to rats, pigs and rabbits, indicating that sheep could be a suitable species for translational coagulation studies. The maximum clot firmness was similar in rabbits and humans, supporting the usefulness of rabbits as a species for examining platelets. The maximum lysis was similar in humans and pigs, confirming the potential usefulness of pigs as an experimental species to study fibrinolytic pathway. STUDY II: Thrombin induced bleedings and death in some rats, which both correlated with the severity of changes in laboratory parameters of DIC. Thrombin increased only IL-6 levels but not other cytokines. In addition, lepirudin prevented thrombin- induced thrombocytopenia. STUDY III: Thrombin (0.42IU/kg/min) induced a haemorrhagic state in sheep, which correlated with the laboratory signs of consumptive coagulopathy. Interestingly, thrombin increased the activity of the coagulation factors V and X and decreased the activity of factors VIII and XIII.

**CONCLUSION:** Protracted intravenous infusion of thrombin in sheep and rats over a period of five hours offers a new experimental model of a bleeding coagulopathy, which can be further used to study isolated effects of thrombin *in vivo*.

# 1. INTRODUCTION

## 1.1. Identification of thrombin

Thrombin, described in 1892 by Alexander Schmidt, was first identified by Buchanan in 1845 [1]. Buchanan reported that the addition of a liquid obtained from a pressed blood-clot to an ascitic fluid, serum or hydrocele fluid, produces a coagulum similar to that which separates spontaneously from blood. Thrombin was then identified as a substance capable of promoting the formation of a fibrous blood clot [1]. The early empirical observations indicated that thrombin can be generated when its precursor (prothrombin) was combined with calcium (lime salts) [2]. Prothrombin was believed to be generated by thrombogen in the presence of thrombokinase (which we today recognise as factor X). Although this historic concept has not proven correct, the link between prothrombin and factor X has been correctly recognised as the prothrombinase complex (factor Xa, factor Va, calcium ions and anionic phospholipid) [3], which catalyzes the conversion of the inactive zymogen prothrombin to the active serine protease thrombin [2].

## 1.2. Evolution of thrombin

Thrombin diverged from the complement factors C1r, C1s or MASP2 in the deuterostome lineage, and this was heralding the onset of further specialisation of defense mechanisms [4]. As complement evolved from developmental proteases, thrombin most likely descended from growth factors. It pre-dated and presumably gave rise to the vitamin K- dependent proteases: factors VIIa, IXa and Xa and protein C [4].

The sequence of the heavy chain of human thrombin is related to the digestive serine proteases trypsin and chymotrypsin with 35% sequence identity and 49% sequence similarity [2]. The structure of thrombin is similar to that of trypsin with regard to its topology, active site geometry and the presence of the critical salt bridge in the active molecule [2].

## 1.3. Biosynthesis of prothrombin

Prothrombin (70 kDa), a glycoprotein with 579 amino acid residues, is produced in the liver parenchymal cells and secreted into the blood [5]. The sequence of human prepro-prothrombin consists of several discrete functional units: a prepro leader sequence, a gamma-carboxyglutamic acid domain, two domains and a carboxy-terminal serine protease domain. Prothrombin undergoes a number of posttranslational modifications prior to its conversion to thrombin. The signal peptide is removed from prepro-prothrombin by signal peptidase following import of the nascent polypeptide into the endoplasmic

*Introduction*

reticulum [2]. The resulting molecule, pro-prothrombin, is then modified by gamma-glutamyl carboxylase, which catalyzes the vitamin K-dependent conversion of glutamate residues to gamma-carboxyglutamate residues [5]. This essential modification confers upon the gamma-carboxyglutamate domain the ability to bind calcium ions and adopt a conformation required for binding to anionic phospholipid surfaces at sites of vascular injury and on activated platelets. Following gamma-glutamyl carboxylation, the propeptide is removed by a furin-like proprotein convertase to generate the amino terminus of the mature zymogen [5]. Following the attachment of N-linked carbohydrate, prothrombin is secreted into the blood where it is found at a concentration of 1.2 mM [2]. Prothrombin is converted to thrombin by the prothrombinase complex consisting of the factor Xa, the cofactor FVa, anionic phospholipids on the surface of activated platelets and calcium ions. Factor Xa cleaves prothrombin to generate meizothrombin, which subsequently is cleaved to liberate thrombin [4].

**1.4. Structure of thrombin**

Thrombin has a molecular weight of 37 kDa. The proteolytically active thrombin molecule is a heterodimer consisting of two polypeptide chains A and B. The light chain A consisting of 36 residues is linked by a single disulfide bond to the heavy chain B with 259 residues that contains three intrachain disulfide bonds [5]. Thrombin is a sodium activated allosteric enzyme [6]. Sodium binding is required for cleavage of fibrinogen, and activation of factors V, VIII and XI. Two allosteric states have been defined that are characterized by the absence and presence of sodium ions, resulting in a slow and a fast form of thrombin [5]. The fast thrombin form cleaves fibrinogen and protease activated receptors and displays procoagulant, prothrombotic, and prosignaling properties. In contrast, the slow form preferentially cleaves protein C, exhibiting more anticoagulant properties [4,5]. The X-ray structure determination of thrombin shows that the molecule can be divided into several functional regions. Although thrombin has an almost neutral isoelectric point, charged residues are clustered, resulting in a pronounced electrostatic field [7]. The catalytic residues are at the edge of a negatively charged surface patch. This acidic region is sandwiched between two positive poles to the active site. The eastern positive patch plays a role in interactions with fibrinogen, fibrin, hirudin, thrombomodulin and thrombin receptor [7]. The northwest patch is the heparin binding site [7].

*Introduction*

## 1.5. Thrombin and genetics

The prothrombin gene is located on the eleventh chromosome (11p11.2) [8]. The congenital Factor II deficiency is an autosomal recessive inherited disorder, which results in a bleeding disorder [9]. Factor II deficiency occurs in approximately 1 in 1–2 million people and is not related to gender or blood type. Mutations occur in a heterozygous, or rarely a homozygous form [8]. More than 40 mutations in prothrombin leading to prothrombin deficiency have been reported, including 35 missense/nonsense and 2 splice site mutations, 4 small deletions, and 1 small insertion [8]. Besides prothrombin deficiencies, dysprothrombinemia characterized by an abnormal function of the molecule, has been reported. Mutations associated with dysprothrombinemia can be divided into two groups: those that produce defects in prothrombin activation and those with defects in the thrombin molecule that is formed. Low prothrombin activity typically prolongs both the activated partial thromboplastin time and prothrombin time [8]. Patients who have defects in the prothrombin gene can present with moderate to severe bleeding symptoms including easy bruising, mucosal bleeding, surgical bleeding, trauma-related bleeding, haemarthroses, and intracranial haemorrhage [10].

## 1.6. Functions of thrombin in coagulation

Thrombin has many functions in the coagulation cascade (Table 1.1, Figure 1.1) [4,11]. The major procoagulant effect, the conversion of fibrinogen to fibrin, is amplified by activation of factor XIII that covalently stabilizes the fibrin clot. Following its activation, factor XIII induces soluble fibrin monomers to interact end-to-end and side-to-side, causing it to become a soluble cross-linked fibrin monomer. Also, the inhibition of fibrinolysis via activation of thrombin-activable fibrinolysis inhibitor (TAFI) and the proteolytic activation of factors V, VIII and XI (Figure 1.1) contribute to the procoagulant activity of thrombin. Regarding the thrombin function as anticoagulant, activation of protein C is highly important. The activation depends on the binding to thrombomodulin, a membrane receptor on endothelial cells [4]. In turn, thrombin is inhibited by thrombomodulin, protein C, heparin cofactor II and antithrombin III with the help of acidic carbohydrates [5]. Because of its dual role in haemostasis thrombin has received much attention in structure-function studies and as a target of anticoagulant therapy.

*Introduction*

| | Thrombin functions in coagulation |
|---|---|
| **Procoagulant properties** | • cleavage of fibrinogen and liberation of fibrinopeptide A and B [5]<br>• activation of factors: V [12], VIII [13], XI [14] and XIII [15]<br>• induction of platelet aggregation, platelet secretion and platelet procoagulant activity [16]<br>• release of adenosine diphosphate from platelets [16]<br>• expression of P-selectin on endothelial cells [17,18]<br>• stimulation of expression of the platelet activating factor (PAF) |
| **Anticoagulant properties** | • binding to thrombomodulin (TM) and activation of protein C<br>• decrease in the binding of von Willebrand factor (vWF) to glycoprotein (GP) Ib [19]<br>• decrease in ristocetin-induced agglutination [19] |
| **Antifibrinolytic properties** | • activation of thrombin-activable fibrinolysis inhibitor (TAFI) [20]<br>• release of the plasminogen activator inhibitor-1 [21] |
| **Fibrinolytic properties** | • release of the tissue plasminogen activator [22] |

**Table 1.1.** Thrombin functions in coagulation.

## 1.7. Pleiotropic functions of thrombin

In addition to the role in haemostasis, thrombin is known to have pleiotropic effects, i.e. it affects the activity of multiple cell types including blood platelets, endothelial cells, vascular smooth muscle cells, monocytes, T lymphocytes and fibroblasts. Thrombin has important role in inflammation and cellular proliferation (Table 1.2, Figure 1.1) [11]. Thrombin modulates multiple processes in the vascular system including vascular permeability, vascular tone, inflammation and neovessel formation. Thrombin also activates numerous cells involved in the inflammatory and reparative responses, including monocytes, T lymphocytes and mast cells, and endothelial cells. It affects leukocyte migration, oedema formation, and other processes related to tissue repair [23]. However, most of these pleiotropic effects of thrombin were documented only in *in vitro* studies (Table 1.2).

### *1.7.1. Protease activated receptors (PARs)*

The protease activated receptors (PARs) are essential in many pleiotropic functions of thrombin. In the activation of platelets and other cells via PARs, thrombin serves as a central effector. PARs are a family of seven-transmembrane G-protein-coupled receptors [24]. Four PARs are currently known. Thrombin activates PAR1, PAR3 and PAR4. PAR2 is not cleaved by thrombin but can be activated by trypsin-like serine proteases.

Interspecies differences in PARs are well known. While human platelets express PAR1 and PAR4 [25] and do not contain PAR3, mice platelets express PAR3 and PAR4 [26,27], but signalling occurs via PAR4 only. Guinea pig platelets have a triple PAR expression pattern: PAR1, PAR2 and PAR3 [27].

*Introduction*

Endothelial cells are considered the main cells mediating vascular effects of PARs [28]. PAR-1 is the major thrombin receptor expressed by endothelial cells, which is up-regulated by thrombin *via* kruppel-like transcription factor 2. Endothelial cells also express PAR-2, PAR-3 and PAR-4. In normal arteries thrombin can induce endothelium-dependent vasorelaxation or direct smooth muscle contraction. Besides the modulation of the vascular tone, thrombin exerts a wide range of effects on endothelial cells among them changes in vascular permeability and induction of endothelial secretory responses [28]. PARs contribute to the pro-inflammatory phenotype observed in endothelial dysfunction and their up-regulation in vascular smooth muscle cells seems to be an important element in the pathogenesis of atherosclerosis and restenosis [28].

The effect of PAR deficiency was examined in a mouse endotoxemia model. Endotoxin-induced thrombocytopenia was not diminished in PAR4 (-/-) mice, suggesting that a mechanism independent of platelet activation by thrombin was sufficient to cause thrombocytopenia and therefore, a role for PAR4 in linking coagulation to inflammation could not be confirmed [29]. Another study has shown that the activation of PAR-2 may not play a pivotal role in endotoxin-induced multi-organ dysfunction in mice [30]. Accordingly, PAR-1 expression was normal in critically ill patients with sepsis [31]. This is in contrast to experimental endotoxemia where the activation of multiple PARs by coagulation proteases enhanced inflammation [32]. A prospective study in 40 healthy men has shown that PAR1 expression is down-regulated on platelets during systemic thrombin formation induced by inflammation. This results in decreased responsiveness to subsequent stimulation of the PAR1 receptor [33].

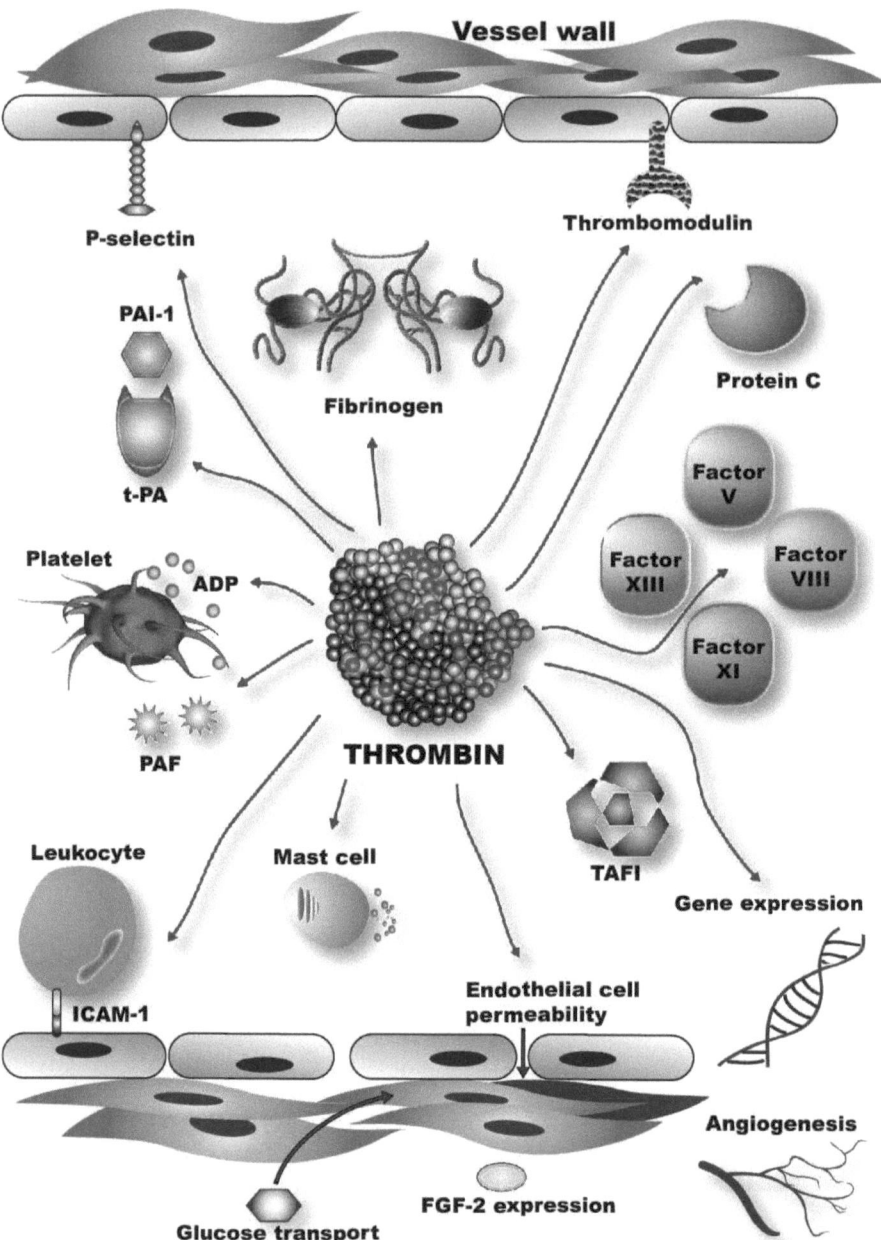

**Figure 1.1.** Multiple functions of thrombin.

*Introduction*

**Pleiotropic functions of thrombin**

| | |
|---|---|
| • endothelial P-selectin expression [34]<br>• endothelial PAF formation [35,36]<br>• CD 40L induced MCP-1, IL6 and IL8 [34]<br>• expression of IL-1beta, TNF-alpha [37], IL-11 [38], IL-10 [39]<br>• PGE-2 formation [40]<br>• mast cell degranulation [41]<br>• leukocyte adherence to endothelial cells via expression of intercellular adhesion molecule-1 (ICAM-1) [42]<br>• endothelial cell activation via PAR-1 and PAR-4 [35,43]<br>• increase of endothelial cell permeability [44]<br>• formation of PDGF and TGFß in platelets [34]<br>• PDGF formation in endothelium [34]<br>• angiogenesis: formation of matrix metalloproteinase (MMP-1 and -2), vascular endothelial growth factor (VEGF), angiopoietin-2 (Ang-2), CD31, and activation of KDR and CXCR2 receptors in human umbilical vein and endothelial cells [45]<br>• gene expression: proto-oncogene c-*fos* [46], endothelin (ET)- 1 [47], growth-regulated oncogene-alpha (GRO-alpha) [45], HOXA10 [43,48], alkaline phosphatase (ALP) [35,49], vascular smooth muscle cell (VSMC) DNA [50], PLA(2) formation [51]<br>• endocytosis of endoglin and type-II TGF-beta receptor and down-regulation of TGF-beta signalling in endothelial cells [52]<br>• glucose transport via Src-p38 MAPK pathway in vascular smooth muscle cells [53]<br>• expression of FGF-2 in vascular smooth muscle cells [50]<br>• activation of p21-activated kinase (PAK) in pulmonary artery smooth muscle cells [54] | IN VITRO |
| • Erk1/2 activation [55] | EX VIVO |
| • MCP-1 formation [43] | IN VIVO |

**Table 1.2.** Pleiotropic functions of thrombin.

### *1.7.2. Thrombin and platelets*

Thrombin is the most potent platelet activator, producing an effect at concentrations lower than those required for activation of the coagulation cascade [56]. Thrombin binds the PAR-1 receptor on the platelet surface, cleaving the receptor, and exposing a tethered ligand, which binds and activates the receptor. At higher concentrations, thrombin also activates PAR-4. Signalling via PAR-4 is available for haemostasis when very high levels of thrombin are generated, thereby providing a protective mechanism in situations where this pathway may contribute to arrest bleeding, such as trauma [56].

Thrombin also binds to the GPIb on the platelet surface [56]. Different experimental approaches conclude that both exosite I and exosite II of thrombin bind to GPIb [57]. However, the pathophysiological relevance of thrombin binding to platelet GPIb is still uncertain, and the key question wheather thrombin binding to GPIb is prothrombotic or antithrombotic remains unanswered yet [57].

*Introduction*

*1.7.3. Thrombin and cancer*

Thrombin exhibits mitogen activity on smooth muscle cells and endothelial cells. Most of the cellular effects elicited by thrombin are mediated through activation and subsequent signal transduction cascades of members of the PAR family. Thrombin activates angiogenesis, a process which is essential in tumor growth and metastasis (Figure 1.1, Table 1.2). The angiogenic and tumor-promoting effect of thrombin can be explained as follows [58]. Thrombin decreases the ability of endothelial cells to attach to basement membrane proteins *via* cyclic adenosine monophosphate, which makes them more mobile. Thrombin also potentiates vascular endothelial growth factor (VEGF) - induced endothelial cell proliferation. This process is accompanied by up-regulation of the expression of VEGF receptors. In addition, thrombin increases the mRNA and protein levels of alpha(v)/beta(3) integrin and it can bind to this receptor [58]. Furthermore, thrombin indirectly up-regulates the transcription of VEGF by inducing the production of reactive oxygen species and the expression of the hypoxia-inducible factor 1 [58].

Thrombin promotes reversible rounding of endothelial cells and increases vascular permeability, resulting in plasma protein leakage and the development of a provisional proangiogenic matrix [23]. By mobilizing adhesion molecules to the cell surface, thrombin enhances adhesion between tumor cells, platelets, endothelial cells, and the extracellular matrix, and contributes to tumor progression. Furthermore, it can trigger the release of growth factors, chemokines and extracellular proteins that promote the proliferation and migration of tumor cells (Table 1.2) [23]. Immobilized thrombin functions as a chemoattractant to endothelial cells by inducing their migration and invasion. Thrombin also facilitates invasion through the basement membrane by activating the collagen type IV degrading enzyme and matrix metalloproteinase 2 [23].

## 1.8. Role of thrombin in disseminated intravascular coagulation (DIC)

Disseminated intravascular coagulation (DIC) is a syndrome of activated coagulation that manifests with concurrent bleeding and/or thrombosis. Patients with DIC have a loss of balance between the clot-promoting and lysing systems *in vivo* [59]. DIC can manifest clinically in different ways from bleeding to thrombosis. Although bleeding is the archetypal physical manifestation in patients with DIC, as a result of reduced platelets and coagulation factors, multiple organ failure is a much more common finding [60]. Morbidity associated with DIC usually results from bleeding, multi organ failure, vascular thrombosis or limb ischemia. DIC is highly relevant for the outcome in patients with sepsis as the presence of DIC increases the risk of mortality beyond that associated with the primary

*Introduction*

disease. Overt DIC has a mortality rate of 50% and represents an urgent medical need [61]. Thrombin generation and release of thrombin into the circulation are central in the initiation of DIC [62]. Tissue factor plays a major part in the initial thrombin formation. Mechanisms responsible for sustaining thrombin generation include: activation of the intrinsic pathway of coagulation, reduction of endogenous anticoagulant factor concentrations, mainly protein C, and increased availability of negatively charged phospholipid surfaces (externalisation of inner cellular membrane leaflet, cellular microparticle formation, circulating lipoproteins) [60]. Tissue factor, expressed on the surface of activated mononuclear cells and endothelial cells, binds and activates factor VII. The tissue factor - factor VIIa complex then activates factor X directly and via factor IX and factor VIII. Simultaneously, physiologic anticoagulants such as antithrombin III, protein S, protein C and tissue factor pathway inhibitor TFPI) are impaired or decreased in concentration [63]. The resulting intravascular formation of fibrin is not balanced by adequate removal of fibrin because endogenous fibrinolysis is suppressed by high plasma levels of plasminogen-activator inhibitor type 1 (PAI-1). The high levels of PAI-1 inhibit plasminogen-activator activity and consequently reduce the rate of formation of plasmin [64]. Dysfunction of endothelial cells further promotes DIC. The manifestation of either thrombotic or bleeding symptoms depend also on genetic and other host-related factors [60].

## 1.9. Animal studies examining effects of thrombin *in vivo*

Several groups have studied the effects of intravenous thrombin infusion in animals (Table 1.3). The effects induced by infusion of thrombin were studied in mice [65-67], rats [68-70], guinea pigs [71], rabbits [72,73], minipigs [74], dogs [75,76] and monkeys [77,78]. When high doses of thrombin (>70U/kg) were administered into the blood stream as a bolus or as a short infusion microthrombi were particularly evident in the lung [71], liver [79], kidney [80], medulla oblongata [77], renal cortex [77], coronary arteries [77] and heart ventricle [75] (LD50=24U/kg [77]).

In contrast, when thrombin was infused slowly at steady-state conditions (0.9-1.6 U/kg/min over 2-5hours), no intravascular clotting but bleedings occurred, which might indicate that without damage of endothelium or alterations in the vessel wall the fibrinolytic and anticoagulant properties of thrombin overweigh [81,82].

Intravenous thrombin infusion caused consumption of clotting factors: Ia, Ib, II,V, VII, VIII [75], IX, X and XII [78], thrombocytopenia [83,84] and a decrease in fibrinogen concentration [85] (Table 1.4). Moreover, thrombin decreased levels of ATIII [86], thrombin antithrombin complexes (TAT) [87], plasminogen activator inhibitor (PAI) [72] and leukocyte count [88]. Simultaneously, thrombin increased the levels of fibrin degradation products

*Introduction*

(FDP) [89], prolonged activated partial thromboplastin time (aPTT) [78,84], prothrombin time [80], thrombin time [74] and thrombin clotting time [85]. Accordingly, thrombin evoked haemolysis [75], increased levels of free haemoglobin [90], histamin and serotonin [73] and resulted in activation of protein C [78] and granulocytosis [88] (Table 1.4).

The cardiorespiratory effects of thrombin were studied in a DIC model in dogs [91], in a thromboembolism model in mice [92], in a model of pulmonary microembolism in guinea pig [71] and in a model of adult respiratory distress syndrome in pigs [74]. Short thrombin infusion (180 U/kg for 20 minutes) resulted in reduction in cardiac output and arterial pressure, an increase in pulmonary artery pressure and alveolar oedema [91]. These symptoms were due to acute pulmonary thromboembolism [91]. Histological examination of lung tissue after thrombin injection showed microthrombi composed of platelet aggregates and fibrin [92]. Accordingly, thrombin caused interstitial and alveolar haemorrhage in the lung [91], increased bronchial resistance [71], pulmonary leucostasis, respiratory insufficiency [74], increased respiratory frequency and respiratory minute volume [91], as well as pulmonary heart disease [77] (Table 1.4).

Interestingly, thrombin infusion also affected blood pressure. Thrombin- induced hypotension and the decrease in blood flow were most likely due to the vasodilation and increased vascular permeability [69,83,93]. Accordingly, infusion of thrombin (3 U/kg) intra-arterially for four hours greatly enlarged the volume of severe vascular disruption and promoted blood-brain barrier leakage of IgG in a model of brain ischemia in rats [94].

| Species | Weight | Dose | Duration of Infusion | Organ pathology | Laboratory parameters | Mortality/ sacrificed | Reference |
|---|---|---|---|---|---|---|---|
| **MOUSE** | 20g-30g | * 1250 U/kg | bolus | pulmonary embolism (at 15 min) | | 80,7% mortality | 65, 66, 67 |
| | | * 1000 U/kg | | | | 68,7% mortality | |
| | | * 750 U/kg | | | | 60% mortality | |
| | | * 800 U/kg | | acute pulmonary embolism | | 90% mortality after 24 h | 95 |
| | | * 3,8-15NIH U/mouse= 160-750 U/kg | | acute pulmonary embolism: microthrombi in the lung | | 100% mortality after 55 min by 15 U | 92 |
| | | *2U/mouse = 100U/kg | | | systemic activation of coagulation system: <br> * ↓ SF (soluble fibrin) <br> * ↓ TAT (thrombin-antithrombin complex) <br> * ↓ ATIII <br> * ↓ leukocyte <br> * ↓ thrombocyte | | 87 |
| **RAT** | 300g | 1,2-1,3 U/min | 15 min -3 h | * glomerular thrombi <br> * 108-120 U during 90 min = renal cortical necrosis | | sacrificed | 68 |
| | 250-300g | 15U/100g + fibronectin | 30 min | Hypotension | * ↓ fibrinogen <br> * ↓ thrombocyte (18-31%) <br> * ↑FDP | 25% mortality | 69 |
| | | 15U/100g + antifibrone | | | * ↓ fibrinogen <br> * ↓ thrombocyte 75% | 87% mortality | |

## Introduction

| Animal | Weight | Dose | Time | Effects | Lab findings | Outcome | Ref |
|---|---|---|---|---|---|---|---|
| RAT | 120-150g | ctin 150-3300 U/kg | | * haemostasis defect on injured veins, but not on injured arteries<br>* platelets agglomeration failure | | | 70 |
| | | | | | * ↓ fibrinogen (39%) after 1h<br>* ↑ fibrinogen (38%) after 24h<br>* resistant for defibrination | Death | 85 |
| GUINEA PIG | | 25 U/kg/min<br><br>8U total<br>10 U/kg/min | 30 min | thrombi in major pulmonary artery<br><br>* bronchial resistance ↑<br>* thrombi in minor pulmonary artery | | 100% mortality | 71 |
| RABBIT | 2,2-3,5 kg | 8,5-38 U/kg<br>LD$_{50}$ = 24 U/kg | 2 min | * hypotension<br>* thrombi: heart ventricle, major vessel | | sacrificed | 77 |
| | 1,8-2,5 kg | 1U/kg/min + 0,5 µg/endotoxin | 60 min | | * ↓ PAI (50%)<br>* ↑ protein C<br>* ↑ APTT (activated partial thromboplastin time) | sacrificed | 72 |
| | 3-4 kg | 75 NIH U in 8 ml | 10s | blood-clot formation after 60 min | * ↓ thrombocyte (90% after 30 min)<br>↑serotonin<br>↑histamine | sacrificed? | 73 |
| | 3-4 kg | 1,25 – 80 IU thrombin/kg/min (thrombin-heparin mixture 3 IU: 1 NIH U) | 5-10 min | thrombin+heparin= without symptoms | * ↓ AT III (10-32 % after 1h) | sacrificed | 86 |
| | | 80-100 IU thrombin/kg/min (thrombin-heparin mixture 3 IU: 1 NIH U) | | | * ↓ AT III (18 % after 1h) | 100% mortality | |
| | 1,5-2kg | 850-900U/100 ml saline | 2h | * kidney necrosis,<br>* fibrin deposit in glomeruli | | 43% mortality during 24 h | 96 |
| | 2,5-3,5kg | 150 NIH U/kg/50ml saline | 20 min | * intravascular fibrin thrombi<br>* alveolar pulmonary oedema<br>* cardiac output ↓<br>* blood pressure↓<br>* pulmonary artery pressure↑ | | | 90 |
| | 2,5-3kg | 2-4 U/ml=2-5,6 ml/min<br>* 2-3 U/min<br><br>*100Utotal | up to death | | * ↑ thrombin clotting time<br>* defibrination | 3U/min = 50% mortality | 85 |
| | 1,6-2,5kg | 120-400U/kg + cortison | 1-1,5h | Without any change in glomeruli | * ↓fibrinogen (32%)<br>* mean fibrinogen consumption = 43-61 mg/kg | 60% mortality | 97 |
| MINIPIG | | 75-150 IE U/kg/h | 3-5 h | * pulmonary pressure ↑<br>* pulmonary leukostasis↑<br>* respiratory insufficiency<br>* saturation ↓ | * ↓ thrombocyte<br>* ↓ leukocyte<br>* DIC<br>* ↑ PTT<br>* ↑ TT (thrombin time) | sacrificed | 74 |
| PIG | 24-48 kg | 250 IU/50 ml saline<br>6,25 IE/Min + ligation of v.cava | 40 min | thrombi in v. cava and v. iliaca | | 8% mortality | 98 |
| DOG | | 500 NIH U/kg | bolus | * major thrombi: right ventricle, major veins,<br>* minor thrombi: lung | * haemolysis (after 30 min)<br>* ↓ factor Ia (100 %)<br>* ↓ factor Ib (67 %)<br>* ↓ factor II (34 %)<br>* ↓ factor V (81 %)<br>* ↓ factor VII (11 %)<br>* ↓ factor VIII (99 %) | sacrificed | 75 |
| | 9-21kg | 50-250 NIH U/kg | | * 35 % pulmonary embolism | * ↓ fibrinogen (20-44 %)<br>* ↓ thrombocyte | 20% mortality | 76 |
| | | 150 NIH U/kg + | | | * ↓ fibrinogen<br>* ↓ thrombocyte | 25% mortality | |

## Introduction

| | | | | | | | |
|---|---|---|---|---|---|---|---|
| **DOG** | | aminocaproic acid | | | | | |
| | 10-15kg | 75 – 250 IU thrombin/kg/min (thrombin-heparin mixture 3 IU: 1 NIH U) | 5-10 min | Without any symptoms | * ↓ AT III (10-33 % after 1h) | sacrificed | 86 |
| | | 2500 IU thrombin/kg/min (thrombin-heparin mixture 5 IU: 1 NIH U) | | * DIC (after 20-40 min) | * ↓ AT III (10-50 % after 1h) | 100% mortality | |
| | | 5000 IU thrombin/kg/min (thrombin-heparin mixture 7 IU: 1 NIH U) | | * DIC (after 20-40 min | * ↓ AT III (10-42 % after 1h) | Death | |
| | 9-22kg | 0,6-15 ml/min/kg * thrombin concentration in blood: 0,02-0,6 U/ml | 10 min | vasodilatation | * ↓ thrombocyte (53%) * ↑ blood flow (35%) | sacrificed | 83 |
| | | 100-150 NIH U/kg | 13 min | microthrombi: - lung - kidney | blood: * thrombocyte↓ * fibrinogen ↓ lung: * thrombocyte↑ * fibrinogen ↑ | | 90 |
| | 22-34kg | 150-180 NIH U/kg | 20 min | * intravascular fibrin thrombi: -lung: interstitial alveolar, perivascular hemorrhage - minor artery <50μm und >50 50μm * ↑respiratory frequency * ↑ respiratory minute volume | After 4 h: * thrombocyte↓ (70 %) * fibrinogen ↓ (67 %) * hematocrit ↑ (28 %) * haemoglobin ↑ (29 %) | 71% mortality after 4h | 91 |
| | 14-23 kg | 75 NIH U/kg | 30 min | * 80% blood flow in kidney *glomerulothrombosis | * ↓ fibrinogen (59%) | | 99 |
| | 35kg | 1-25 NIH U/ml in the renal artery * concentration in blood: 0,01-0,05 NIH U/ml | | * renal blood flow↓ 10-50% (vasoconstriction?) * femoral blood flow ↑ 100-200% | | | 93 |
| | 13-16 kg | 70 NIH U/kg | 30 min | * DIC * accumulation of fibrin in glomeruli | * ↓ fibrinogen (70-80 % after 60-120 min) * factor II no change * ↓ factor V (80-90 %after 30-60 min) * factor VII no change * ↓ factor VIII (85-90 %) * ↓ thrombocyte * haemolysis (30 min-3 h) in 50% animals * ↑ phrothrombin time * ↑ partial thromboplastin time | sacrificed | 80 |
| | 9,5-27kg | 70NIH U/kg/100ml saline | 30 min | respiratory stridor | * ↓ factor V (56 % after 30-60 min) * ↓ factor VIII (25 %) * ↓ thrombocyte (66%) * ↓ leukocyte (34%) * haemolysis * granulocytosis * ↑ FDP | 30% mortality | 88 |
| | 17-26kg | 310 NIH U/kg | 30 min | | * ↓ thrombocyte * ↓ fibrinogen * ↑ hematokrit | sacrificed | 79 |

*Introduction*

| | | | | | | |
|---|---|---|---|---|---|---|
| **DOG** | | 310 NIH U/kg + AMCA (tranexamic acid) | | * respiratory insufficiency<br>* fibrin thrombi in lung and liver<br>* pulmonary oedema | | 43% mortality |
| | | 310 NIH U/kg | 30 min | * microemboli in lung,<br>* pulmonary oedema | * ↓ thrombocyte<br>* ↓ fibrinogen | Sacrificed | 100 |
| | 17-28kg | 150 NIH U/kg | 30 min | * blood pressure↓<br>* pulmonary artery pressure↑<br>* cardiac output ↓<br>* pulmonary oedema+minor thrombi | * ↑ heart lymph flow (81%)<br>* ↑hematocrit<br>* ↓ ATT (aspartate aminotransferase) in heart lymph | Sacrificed | 101 |
| | 7-12kg | 40 NIH U/min | 125 min | | * ↑ FDP (fibrinogen degradation products)<br>* ↑ thrombin clotting time | | 89 |
| | 8-10kg | 200 U total | up to death | | * ↓ ATIII<br>* ↓ fibrinogen (60%)<br>* ↓ thrombocyte (20%) | | 85 |
| | | 70U/kg/h | 2h | 1U/ml/min/kg enough to cause DIC | * ↓ thrombocyte<br>* ↓ fibrinogen<br>* ↓ prothrombin time | | 82 |
| **MONKEY** | 3,2-4,2 kg | 166-275U/kg = lethal dose | bolus | * cor pulmonale<br>* hypotension<br>* apnoea,<br>* microthrombi: lung, liver, kidney, medulla, renal cortex, coronary artery, | * ↓ thrombocyte 58-82%<br>* ↓ fibrinogen (42-61%) | 100 % mortality after minutes | 77 |
| | 5,9-6,7kg | 1-2.5µg/kg/min | 10 min | | * ↑ APTT (greater in animals with aterogenic diet in comparison with control group)<br>* ↑ APC (activated protein C)<br>* ↓ thrombocyte (15%)<br>* ↓ fibrinogen (35%)<br>* ↓ factor V (40-50 % after ,30-60 min)<br>* ↓ factor VIII (60-70 %)<br>* ↓ factor IX, X, XII (30%)<br>* ↓ protein C (15%) | | 78 |

**Table 1.3.** Summary of animal studies examining thrombin effects *in vivo* after intravenous thrombin infusion.

*Introduction*

| SUMMARY: thrombin effects *in vivo* after intravenous infusion in animals ||
|---|---|
| **Organ pathology** | **Laboratory Parameters** |
| **Lung:**<br>• pulmonary embolism: microthrombi [a,c,d,g,h]<br>• interstitial, alveolar or perivascular haemorrhage [g]<br>• alveolar pulmonary oedema [d,g]<br>• ↑ bronchial resistance [c]<br>• ↑ pulmonary artery pressure [e]<br>• ↑ pulmonary leucostasis [e]<br>• respiratory insufficiency [e,g]<br>• ↑ respiratory frequency [g]<br>• ↑ respiratory minute volume [g]<br>• respiratory stridor [g]<br>**Kidney:**<br>• glomerular thrombi [b,d,g,h]<br>• renal cortical necrosis [b]<br>• ↓ renal blood flow (vasoconstriction) [g]<br>**Vessels:**<br>• hypotension [b,d,h]<br>• vasodilatation [g]<br>• thrombi in v. cava and iliac vein [f]<br>• ↑ femoral blood flow [g]<br>• ↓ oxygen saturation [e]<br>**Heart:**<br>• ↓ cardiac output [d,g]<br>• ↓ blood pressure [d,g]<br>• thrombi in ventricle [d,g]<br>• cor pulmonale [h]<br>• ↑ heart lymph flow [g]<br>**Microthrombi:**<br>• lung: deposition of platelets and fibrinogen [a,c,d]<br>• liver [e]<br>• kidney [d]<br>• medulla [e]<br>• renal cortex [e]<br>• coronary artery [e]<br>• heart ventricle [d]<br>• v. cava and v. Iliac [f] | **Blood:**<br>DIC<br>HEMOLYSIS<br><br>**COAGULATION MARKERS**<br><br>• ↑ FDP (fibrin degradation products) [b,d]<br>• ↑ APTT (activated partial thromboplastin time) [h,d]<br>• ↑ prothrombin time [g]<br>• ↑ thrombin clotting time [d, g]<br>• ↑ TT (thrombin time) [e]<br>• ↑ bleeding time of injured veins, but not of injured arteries [b]<br>• ↓ coagulation factors: Ia [g], Ib [g], II [g], V [g], VII [g], VIII [g], IX [h], X [h], XII [h]<br>• ↓ SF (soluble fibrin) [a]<br>• ↓ fibrinogen [b,d,g,h]<br>• ↓ TAT (thrombin-antithrombin complex) [a]<br>• ↓ ATIII [a,d,g]<br>• ↓ platelets [a,b,e,g,h]<br>• ↓ PAI [d]<br>• ↑ APC (activated protein C) [h]<br><br>**GLOBAL MARKERS**<br><br>• ↑ serotonin [d]<br>• ↑ histamine [d]<br>• ↑ hematocrit [g]<br>• ↑ free haemoglobin [g]<br>• ↑ granulocytes [g] |

**Table 1.3.** Changes in organ functions and laboratory parameters after intravenous thrombin infusion in animals: a-mouse, b-rat, c-guinea pig, d-rabbit, e-minipig, f- pig, g-dog, h-monkey.

## 1.10. Use of thrombin as a therapeutic

The use of thrombin as a topical agent for the treatment of surface bleeding dates from the 1930s [102]. Today, thrombin is frequently used to stop residual bleeding in surgery, especially in cardiovascular surgery and in the treatment of pseudoaneurysms. In the latter case thrombin is injected directly into the aneurysm resulting in the clotting of blood and preventing the rupture of the vessel [102]. The most common industrial fibrin sealant consists of fibrinogen and thrombin. Both components are obtained by fractionation of plasma. The fibrinogen concentrate is usually obtained by precipitation methods from which it is further purified. Thrombin is produced following activation of a partially purified human prothrombin fraction to thrombin, followed by further purification by chromatography [102]. For research purposes human thrombin can be obtained from the thrombin syringe of the fibrin sealant kits.

Recombinant human thrombin is used for therapeutic use minor bleeding from capillaries and small venules is accessible or control of bleeding by standard surgical techniques such as ligature or cautery is ineffective [103].

## 1.11. Use of thrombin inhibitors as a therapeutic

Antithrombotics block the thrombin actions by binding to any of its three enzymatic sites: the active or primary binding site (catalytic site), responsible for thrombin's main activities, the exosite-1, the fibrin recognition site that ensures substrates are bound in proper orientation, or the exosite-2, the binding site for thrombin to indirect thrombin inhibitors i.e., unfractionated heparin (UFH) and low molecular weight heparin (LMWH) [104,105]. Indirect thrombin inhibitors (UFH and LMWH) can inhibit circulating thrombin but cannot inhibit fibrin-bound thrombin. LMWHs (e.g., enoxaparin and dalteparin) and UFH bind to antithrombin and then access exosite-2 to inhibit thrombin's actions [106]. When thrombin is already bound to fibrin at exosite-1, UFH and LMWHs can no longer inhibit thrombin [104].

Direct thrombin inhibitors are small molecules that inhibit thrombin directly and independently from anthithrombin by binding to its active catalytic site and/or its exosite and can inhibit both fibrin/clot bound and free circulating thrombin [106]. Four direct thrombin inhibitors are currently used: - bivalirudin (bivalent binding to the catalytic site and exosite 1 site of thrombin leading to reversible inhibition), hirudin or its recombinant - lepirudin (bivalent binding to the catalytic site and exosite 1 site of thrombin leading to irreversible inhibition), argatroban (univalent binding to the catalytic site of thrombin leading to reversible inhibition), and dabigatran (univalent binding to the catalytic site of thrombin, leading to reversible inhibition) [107].

## 2. RATIONALE AND STUDY AIMS

The complexity of thrombin functions have captured the interest of many researchers and earned this enzyme a dominant place in clotting factor research. Although several decades of research on thrombin functions have provided a framework for understanding the biology of thrombin, studies are still needed to further characterise the functions of thrombin in disease. An example of a disorder where thrombin release plays a central role is disseminated intravascular coagulation (DIC) [108]. DIC is highly relevant to the outcome in patients with sepsis as the presence of DIC increases the risk of mortality beyond that associated with the primary disease. Overt DIC has a mortality rate of 50% and represents an urgent medical need [61]. Therefore, the early detection and treatment as well as identification of biomarkers are goals for the scientific community working on this topic. Accordingly, the International Society of Thrombosis and Haemostasis recommended to perform research in order to facilitate early detection of DIC with emphasis on recognising a non-overt stage [60]. As investigations with regard to early pathophysiological changes in DIC are difficult, animal models of DIC are needed. Although several groups have studied the effects of intravenous thrombin infusion in animals in order to establish a model to study thrombin-induced thromboembolism or thrombosis, in most instances thrombin infusion did not exceed one hour or was a bolus injection. This short period of thrombin infusion is not adequate to study consumptiv coagulopathy, which mostly develops over many days. On the other side, the relevance of animal models to human health is often questioned because of differences between species [109]. The lack of concordance between animal experiments and clinical trials has been reported and may be due to the failure of animal models to adequately represent human disease [109]. In respect to translational research it is relevant which species are comparable to human.

*Aims*

**In this respect we aimed to:**
- perform a cross-species comparison of thrombelastographic blood properties with and without thrombin stimulation of blood from human, rat, sheep, pig and rabbit in order to characterise the species, which mimics the coagulation profile in human most adequately.
- establish rodent and non-rodent models of protracted intravenous thrombin infusion over five hours at steady state conditions, which does not lead to lethal outcome.
- investigate interspecies differences in the biological effects of thrombin, including its role in inflammation.
- study thrombin antagonists in a model of continuous thrombin infusion.

# 3. METHODS

## 3.1. Design of studies

The studies were performed in accordance with the institutional guidance of the Ethics Committee of the Medical University of Vienna and with the Ethics Committee and Government on animal experimentation of Austria. Volunteers provided written informed consent for blood sampling.

### 3.1.1. STUDY I: Interspecies differences in coagulation profile with and without thrombin stimulation

Differences in the coagulation profile with and without thrombin stimulation *in vitro* were compared between five species. The effects of thrombin at doses of 0.0002-1 IU were studied with thromboelastometry. Tubes with 3.8% citrate, heparin or EDTA (BD Vacutainer; Becton Dickinson) were used for blood collection. Blood samples were obtained using a 21-gauge needle. Human venous blood was collected from an antecubital vein. In sheep (female Austrian mountain sheep, Department of Biomedical Research, Himberg, Austria) the jugular vein was used for blood collection, an ear vein was punctured in pigs (Austrian Landrace pig, Veterinary University of Vienna) and rabbits (New Zealand White, Charles River Laboratories, MA, USA). Blood from rats (male Sprague Dawley rats, Department of Biomedical Research, Himberg, Austria) was obtained by terminal heart puncture.

### 3.1.2. STUDY II: A rat model of thrombin – induced consumption coagulopathy

Our pilot experiments performed in Wistar rats showed that prolonged anaesthesia with isoflurane provokes hypotension and multiple organ failure in Wistar rats but not in Sprague Dawley rats [110], which confirmed previous findings on rat strain differences in drug metabolism and effects [111,112]. Therefore, we performed this experiment in male Sprague Dawley rats (Him:OFA/SPF; Biomedical Center Himberg, Austria; n=38) weighing 300-400g. Rats received a standard diet and water *ad libitum* and were housed in rooms maintained at 22-24°C during a 12-h cycle of light and dark. Rats were anesthetized with intraperitoneal injection of ketamine (100mg/kg) (Ketanest, Pfizer, Vienna, Austria) and xylazine (5mg/kg) (Rompun, Bayer, Vienna, Austria) and were subsequently intubated with a silastic cannula. Anaesthesia was sustained with a continuous infusion of fentanyl (0.12mg/kg/h) and ketamine (20mg/kg/h). Rats were ventilated with an air/oxygen (0.8L/1.5L) mixture under 15mmHg pressure. Thrombin (Tissucol Duo Quick, BAXTER

*Methods*

AG, Vienna, Austria) was infused through the lateral caudal vein of the tail with the use of a permanent intravenous catheter over a period of five hours (Infusomat: flow rate 2 ml/h; Venflon, 24 G/19 mm). Blood samples were collected: at baseline (sublingual vein), at 5 (immediately after the end of thrombin infusion) or 24 hours (heart puncture). In animals, which did not survive blood was drawn upon death. Anal temperature was recorded with the thermistor and was maintained at 37-38°C by applying infrared light. Vital parameters were measured before and during intravenous thrombin infusion. At the end of the experiment (5h in the dose escalation study or 24h in the dose verification study), rats were sacrificed and a complete autopsy was performed. The study consisted of three parts: dose escalation, dose verification and a parallel group study to investigate whether thrombin effects can be antagonised by concomitant infusion of lepirudin.

### 3.1.2.1. Part I: *dose escalation*

The primary objective of the dose escalation study was to find thrombin doses inducing changes in laboratory parameters of DIC. The secondary aims of the dose escalation study were to find 1) the lowest observed adverse effect level (*LOAEL;* the lowest thrombin dose causing clinical symptoms of DIC or changes in laboratory parameters of DIC), 2) the no observed adverse effect level (*NOAEL*; a thrombin dose, which is tolerated by the animal without any laboratory changes or evidence of organ dysfunction) and 3) the lethal dose. The starting dose (the highest infusion rate) was selected based on data of two previously published models of thrombin- induced DIC [81,82]. The starting dose was subsequently reduced. Three animals were challenged per dose group (N=3x6) and three rats served as a control group. Animals in the control group received physiologic saline solution.

### 3.1.2.2. Part II: *dose verification*

In order to verify whether thrombin at the no observed adverse effect level (*NOAEL*) can alter animal's behaviour after anaesthesia or cause changes in laboratory parameters after the end of the infusion, thrombin was administered to five additional rats. Two animals were sacrificed immediately after the end of thrombin infusion and three animals were observed for 24 hours and subsequently sacrificed.

### 3.1.2.3. Part III: *lepirudin vs. placebo*

To prove the concept that the effects of thrombin could be antagonised by lepirudin we performed an additional experiment in twelve rats. We were particularly interested whether

*Methods*

clinical symptoms of DIC could be prevented by lepirudin. Therefore, we have chosen the thrombin dose causing bleedings in all animals per group in the dose escalation study (0.3 U/kg/min). All animals received thrombin (0.3 U/kg/min); six of them received lepirudin (cumulative dose 1.5mg) and another six rat's placebo. Both infusions (thrombin/lepirudin or thrombin/placebo) were administered through contra-lateral veins and were started and ended simultaneously.

### 3.1.3. STUDY III: An ovine model of thrombin – induced consumption coagulopathy

Austrian Mountain Sheep (Biomedical Center Himberg, Austria; n=8) weighing 70-80kg received a standard diet and water *ad libitum*. Sheep were housed in rooms maintained at 22-24°C during a 12-h cycle of light and dark. Thrombin was infused through the ear vein with the use of a permanent intravenous catheter over a period of five hours (Infusomat: flow rate 10ml/h; Venflon, 20G/1x30mm). Animals received continuous volume substitution (10mL/h; physiologic saline 0.9%). To avoid influence of anaesthesia on changes in laboratory parameters sheep were neither sedated nor anaesthetised during infusion of thrombin. The study consisted of two parts: dose escalation and dose verification. Blood was drawn through the jugular vein. Samples were collected: at baseline, at 5 (immediately after the end of thrombin infusion), 24, 48 and 72 hours. In the dose verification study blood samples were additionally collected at 1, 2, 3 and 4 hours.

#### 3.1.3.1. Part I: *dose escalation*

The primary objective of the dose escalation study was to find thrombin doses inducing changes in laboratory parameters of DIC. The secondary aims of the dose escalation study were to find 1) the lowest observed adverse effect level (*LOAEL;* the lowest thrombin dose causing clinical symptoms of DIC or changes in laboratory parameters of DIC) and 2) the no observed adverse effect level (*NOAEL*; a thrombin dose, which is tolerated by the animal without any laboratory changes or evidence of organ dysfunction). Two to three subsequent doses of thrombin were tested in each animal (eleven thrombin doses + three control experiments with physiologic saline solution; n=14 experiments). The wash out period was one week.

*Methods*

### 3.1.3.2. Part II: *dose verification*

In the dose verification study thrombin or 0.9% saline solution were administered in three additional animals in a cross over design with a minimum wash out period of one week. To investigate the effects of thrombin in a multiple dose study, one sheep was challenged with thrombin twice. At the end of the experiment (day 8) animals were sacrificed and a complete autopsy was performed.

### 3.2. Modified Rotation Thromboelastometry Analyzer (ROTEM)

The ROTEM, Rotation Thromboelastometry Analyser (Pentapharm, Munich, Germany) gives a graphic representation of clot formation and subsequent lysis. Blood is incubated at 37°C in a heated cup. As fibrin forms between the cup and the pin, the impedance of the rotation of the pin is detected and the trace is generated [113]. The whole blood samples were collected into 3.8% sodium citrate tubes. Measurements were performed within 1 hour after blood sampling. Before running the assay, citrated blood samples were recalcified with 20µl of 0.2 M $CaCl_2$ (Start-TEM) and the NATEM test (a test without any activator = Non-Activated TEM) was started [114]. The following parameters were analyzed: the clotting time (CT), the clot formation time (CFT), the maximum clot firmness (MCF), the maximum lysis (ML) and the alpha angle (alp). The clotting time (CT) characterises the period from analysis start until the start of clot formation. The clot formation time (CFT) describes the subsequent period until the amplitude of 20 mm is reached. The CT and CFT represent the activation and dynamics of clot formation [115] and are sensitive to thrombin generation during endotoxemia [114] as well as anticoagulants used for the treatment of DIC [116]. The maximum lysis (ML) represents the maximum fibrinolysis detected during the analysis [115]. The maximum clot firmness (MCF) gives information about the clot strength and stability. MCF is largely dependent on fibrinogen and platelets and describes platelet function [117,118].

### 3.3. Endogenous thrombin potential (ETP)

The endogenous thrombin potential (ETP) was measured with the Technothrombin fluorogenic assay (Technoclone Vienna, Austria). Technothrombin is a thrombin generation assay based on the monitoring of the formation of thrombin in platelet poor plasma by means of a fluorogenic substrate upon activation of the coagulation cascade by tissue factor (low concentration of phospholipid micelles containing 17.9 pM of recombinant human tissue factor in Tris-Hepes-NaCl buffer) [119]. The reaction was monitored by use of the FLx 800™ TC Fluorometer (BioTek Instruments GmbH, Bad

Friedrichshall, Germany). Readings from the fluorometer were automatically recorded and calculated by Thrombin TGA Evaluation Software (Technoclone, Vienna, Austria).

### 3.4. Platelet Function Analyzer (PFA-100)

The PFA-100 (Dade Behring, Marburg, Germany) was used for measuring platelet function under high shear rates (5000-6000$s^{-1}$). Blood samples collected in 3.8% sodium citrate were used. The PFA-100 measures the time required for occlusion of the aperture by platelet plugs, which is defined as closure time (CT) [120]. The instrument aspirates a blood sample under constant vacuum from the sample reservoir through a capillary and a microscopic aperture (147 μm) cut into the membrane, which leads to high shear induced platelet plug formation. We used cartridges coated with collagen/adenosine diphosphate (CADP) [121].

### 3.5. Impedance Aggregometry

Whole blood aggregation was determined using Multiple Electrode Aggregometry (MEA) on a new generation impedance aggregometer (Multiplate Analyzer, Dynabyte Medical, Munich, Germany) [122]. The system detects the electrical impedance change due to the adhesion and aggregation of platelets on two independent electrode-set surfaces in the test cuvette. We used adenosine diphosphate (ADP; 6.4μM), thrombin receptor-activating peptide (TRAP-6; 30μM) and collagen (3.2μg/ml) as agonists. A 1:2 dilution of whole blood anticoagulated with hirudin and 0.9% NaCl was stirred at 37°C for 3 min in the test cuvettes, ADP, TRAP-6 or collagen were added and the increase in electrical impedance was recorded continuously for 6 min. The mean values of the 2 independent determinations are expressed as the area under the curve of the aggregation tracing (AUC) [123].

### 3.6. Von Willebrand Factor-Ristocetin Cofactor Activity (vWF:RICO)

The vWF:RICO test measuring plasma von Willebrand factor activity was performed by use of turbidometry (Dade Behring; Marburg, Germany) according to the manufacturer's instruction [124].

*Methods*

## 3.7. Two-dimensional electrophoresis (2-DE)

Proteome analysis by two-dimensional electrophoresis (2-DE) was performed on plasma samples from the time points 0, 5, 24, 48 and 72h from animals receiving 125U/kg of thrombin and in control animals. Patterns were compared between controls and treated animals. 2-DE separates proteins in the first dimension according to their charge (isoelectric point) and in the second based on their molecular mass. This combination allows seeing single proteins and/or protein subunits and obtaining high resolution spot patterns. In the applied latest staining technology (2D-DIGE), protein detection relies on pre-electrophoretic minimal labelling of the proteins by fluorescent CyDyes, which permits detection of up to three samples per gel with high sensitivity [125]. Electrophoretic separation was performed according to published protocols [126] in non-linear gradients of pH 4-10 in the presence of urea and CHAPS, followed by SDS-PAGE in 10-15 % T gradient gels. Three different plasma samples were pre-labelled with CyDyes (GE Healthcare Life Sciences, Munich, Germany) and after electrophoretic separation scanned on a Typhoon 9400 and evaluated with DeCyder software. 2-DE was performed on plasma samples, which had been supplemented with protease inhibitors (Mini Complete, Roche Diagnostics GmbH, Penzberg, Germany). Samples from three treated animals and three control animals were investigated at all time points.

## 3.8. Mass spectrometric analysis (MS)

Proteins were identified based on their characteristic peptide pattern obtained after tryptic cleavage and separation according to their size/charge ratio by mass spectrometric analysis (matrix assisted laser desorption ionization tandem time of flight, MALDI-TOF/TOF). 2D-DIGE gels were post-stained with silver, spots of interest were cut and proteins in the obtained gel plugs tryptically digested. The resulting peptide mixtures were analysed by MALDI-TOF/TOF (either on an Ultraflex II, Bruker Daltonics, Bremen, Germany, or an Applied Biosystems 4800 Proteomics Analyzer, Foster City, CA, USA). Proteins were identified by database searches as described [127,128] using the UniProt Knowledgebase Release 15.15 (consisting of UniProtKB/Swiss-Prot Release 57.15 and UniProtKB/TrEMBL Release 40.15, both of 02-Mar-2010).

## 3.9. Other laboratory assays

Fibrinogen concentration, prothrombin time (PT), thrombin time (TT) and activated partial thromboplastin time (aPTT; Diagnostica Stago, Roche, Vienna, Austria) were measured using the KC10 Coagulometer (Amelung GmbH, Lemgo, Germany). The

*Methods*

fibrinogen concentration was measured using the Clauss method, in which human thrombin (70 NIH U/ml) is added to diluted citrated plasma [129]. In the presence of excess of thrombin, the coagulation time is inversely proportional to the fibrinogen concentration. A standard of known concentration is used to generate a standard curve, from which concentrations of fibrinogen are deduced. Prothrombin time was measured with the Normotest according to the manufacturer's instructions (Technoclone, Vienna, Austria). The reagent, which contains rabbit brain thromboplastin and adsorbed bovine plasma (source of factor V and fibrinogen) is added to citrated plasma and the coagulation time is measured until clot formation. The coagulation activity is expressed as percentage of normal value of an adult population. The activated partial thromboplastin time (aPTT) was determined according to the Langdell method [130]. Determination of aPTT involves recalcification of plasma in the presence of a standardized amount of cephalin (platelet substitute from rabbit cerebral tissues) and source factor (Kieselgur). The time is measured from the addition of calcium ions to the formation of clot. D-dimer was measured with the two different methods: the Latex Photometric Immunoassay (Amelung GmbH, Lemgo, Germany) and the D-dimer ELISA kit with cross-reactivity to rat according to the manufacturer's instructions (Diagnostica Stago, Germany). However, all results obtained with D-dimer ELISA kit were below the detection limit. Platelet counts, white blood cell counts and red blood cell counts were quantified with an Abbott-Cell-Dyn counter 3500 (Abbott Diagnostic Division, Vienna, Austria). Alanine amino transferase (ALT), aspartate amino transferase (AST), lactate dehydrogenase (LDH), creatinine, blood urea nitrogen (BUN) and glucose levels were measured by use of Hitachi Automatic Analyzer 904 (Böhringer Mannheim, Germany). Lactate and pH values were measured by use of an ABL800 FLEX blood gas analyzer (Drott Medizintechnik GmbH, Vienna, Austria). The activity of coagulation factors V, X and XI (Siemens, Vienna, Austria), VIII and XIII (Technoclone, Vienna, Austria) were measured by use of the KC10 Coagulometer (Amelung GmbH, Lemgo, Germany) according to the manufacturer instructions. To investigate whether thrombin could affect the sensitivity of the factor X assay, an additional experiment was performed: factor X deficient plasma was mixed 1:1 with pooled plasma and subsequently incubated with 10 different concentrations of thrombin (0.6; 0.2; 0.06; 0.02; 0.006; 0.002; 0.0006; 0.0002; 0.00006 and 0.00002 IU/ml). Afterwards the assay was run.

*Methods*

## 3.10. Measurement of the expression of MCP-1, IL-6, TNF-alpha and IL-10

Enzyme-linked immunosorbant assays of rat monocyte chemotactic protein 1 (MCP-1; Biotrak,GE Healthcare, Austria), IL-6, IL-10 and TNF alpha (R&D Systems, Biomedica, Vienna, Austria) were performed according to the manufacturer's instructions. The intra-assay variability for each test was as follow: MCP-1 <10%, IL-6 7-10%, TNF-alpha 8.8-9.7%, IL-10 7.3-9.9% (according to the manufacturer's information).

## 3.11. Tissue histology

The liver, kidney, lung, spleen, brain and heart of rats and sheep were obtained for histopathological investigations. Perfusion with normal saline followed by 10% neutral buffered formalin was performed. Specimens were embedded in paraffin and stained with two different techniques: 1) hematoxylin and eosin for detection of bleeding or oedema [131] and 2) the Masson trichrome stain for detection of thrombi in the vasculature [132].

## 3.12 Data analysis

### 3.12.1 STUDY I: Interspecies differences in coagulation profile with and without thrombin stimulation

Species differences are mostly presented by descriptive statistics. Data are expressed as mean of six determinations and the standard error of mean (SEM) or median and the range. Non parametric statistics were applied. Statistical comparisons were performed with the Friedman ANOVA, repeated measures ANOVA, the Kruskal-Wallis test, the Wilcoxon signed rank test for *post hoc* comparisons and paired Wilcoxon test. A two-tailed P-value of <0.0125 was considered significant to correct for multiple comparisons between humans and other species for the primary outcome parameter (CT+CFT in ROTEM). All other p values provided are exploratory only.

### 3.12.2. STUDY II: A rat model of thrombin – induced consumption coagulopathy

Statistical comparisons were performed with the paired Wilcoxon test, the Mann Whitney-U test, $\chi^2$ test or Spearman rank correlation test as appropriate. An exact two-sided P-value of <0.05 was considered significant. Data are expressed as median and interquartile range (IQ). As this study was aimed to establish a new experimental model, we did not have a good estimate for the effect size. Hence, we could not calculate any sample size based on a known effect size. For the dose escalation study we assumed a typical number of three animals per group would be sufficient. To be able to demonstrate effects of lepirudin, we calculated that we would need six subjects per group.

*Methods*

### 3.12.3 STUDY III: An ovine model of thrombin – induced consumption coagulopathy

Statistical comparisons were performed with the t-test, paired t-test, one way ANOVA, $\chi^2$ test or Pearson rank correlation test as appropriate. An exact two-sided P-value of <0.05 was considered significant. Data are expressed as mean and standard error of mean (SEM). As this study was aimed to establish a new experimental model, we did not have a good estimate for the effect size. Hence, we could not calculate any sample size based on a known effect size. For the dose escalation study we assumed that one animal per dose would be sufficient. For the dose verification study we assumed a number typical for large animals (n=3 per group).

All statistical calculations were performed using commercially available statistical software (SPSS Version 18.0; Chicago, USA).

# 4. RESULTS

## 4.1. STUDY I: Interspecies differences in coagulation profile with and without thrombin stimulation

### 4.1.1 Interspecies differences measured by ROTEM

The clotting time without thrombin stimulation in humans (mean 595s) was 3 fold longer than in rats (207s) (p=0.001) and 2.5 fold longer than in rabbits (240s) and pigs (244s) (p<0.05) (Figure 2.1A; Table 2.1). The clotting time without thrombin stimulation and the sum of the clotting time and the clot formation time (CT+CFT) were comparable in humans and sheep (Figure 2.1B; Table 2.1).

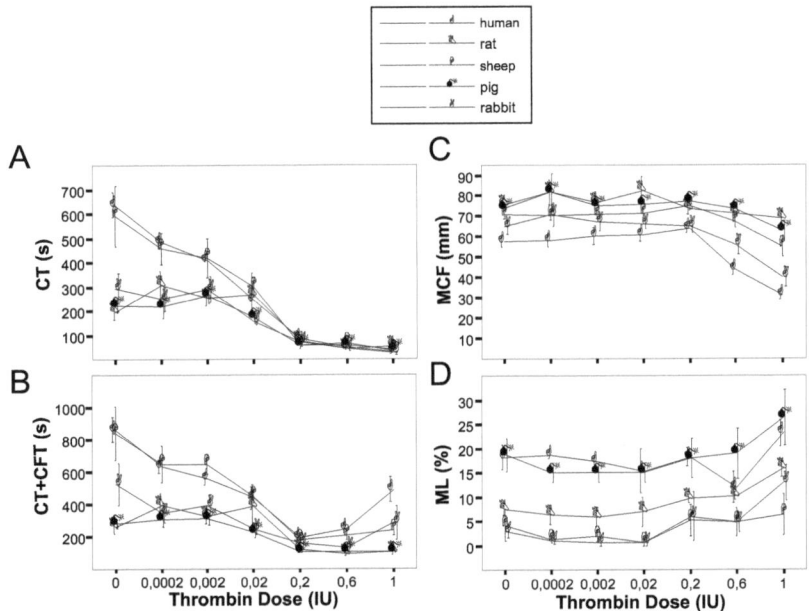

**Figure 2.1.** The effect of thrombin stimulation on A) clotting time (CT), B) sum of clotting time and clot formation time (CT+CFT), C) maximal clot firmness (MCF) and D) maximal lysis (ML) in different species. Data are presented as mean ± SEM. Thrombin concentration is expressed in international units (IU)/300µl blood.

*Results*

|  | CT (s) | CFT (s) | CT+CFT (s) | MCF (mm) | ML (%) |
|---|---|---|---|---|---|
| **Human** | 595 (476-901) | 200 (104-436) | 733 (642-1197) | 58 (49-65) | 21 (2-24) |
| **Rat** | 207 (63-352)*** | 55 (35-97)*** | 266 (102-449)** | 75 (70-81)*** | 8 (3-13)** |
| **Sheep** | 494 (344-1431) | 182 (143-532) | 685 (503-1963) | 72 (61-77)*** | 2 (0-26)*** |
| **Pig** | 244 (146-296)** | 52 (30-84)** | 298 (176-349)** | 74 (68-79)*** | 17 (12-31) |
| **Rabbit** | 240 (130-613)* | 153 (72-751) | 396 (247-1364) | 64 (48-76) | 2 (0-12)*** |

**Table 2.1.** Comparison of the rotation thromboelastometry parameters between species at baseline. Data are presented as median and range. CT=clotting time, CFT=clot formation time, MCF=maximum clot firmness, ML=maximum lysis; *p<0.05; **p<0.01; ***p<0.001 vs. human.

Thrombin shortened the clotting time (CT) with the half maximal effective concentration ($EC_{50}$) of 0.01 IU in humans, 0.02 IU in sheep, 0.03 IU in rabbits, 0.05 IU in pigs and 0.1 IU in rats (Figure 2.2).

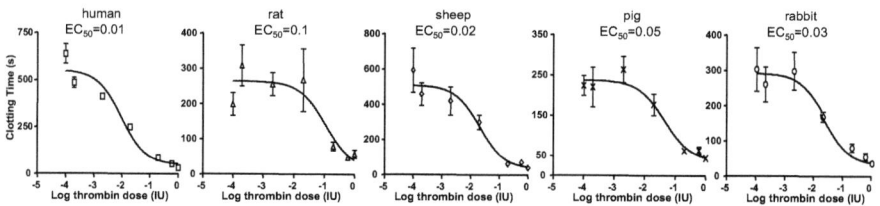

**Figure 2.2.** Concentration-response curves of thrombin on clotting time in different species. ED50=effective thrombin dose that is required for a 50% decrease in clotting time (CT). The X axis is given as a logarithmic scale.

Even the lowest thrombin dose of 0.0002 IU shortened the clotting time by 25% in humans and sheep (Figure 2.1A). A thrombin dose of 0.02 IU decreased the clotting time by 90% as compared to the control in humans and sheep (p<0.05). In rats, pigs and rabbits, 0.2 IU of thrombin was required to shorten the clotting time (p<0.05), which was a 100-fold higher dose of thrombin as compared to humans and sheep. An increase in thrombin dose greater than 0.2 IU did not have a significant additional effect on clotting time in all species.

Maximum clot firmness (MCF) without thrombin stimulation was similar in rabbits (64 mm) and humans (58 mm) (Figure 2.1C). The MCF without thrombin stimulation was in the same range in rats, sheep and pigs (72-75 mm) (Figure 2.1C).

A thrombin dose of 0.06 IU caused a 20% decrease in the MCF in humans and rabbits (p<0.05). One IU of thrombin caused a reduction in MCF by 45% in humans

*Results*

(p=0.004) and 35% in rabbits (p=0.02). Thrombin stimulation did not alter the MCF in rats, sheep and pigs (Figure 2.1C).

The median maximum lysis (ML) without thrombin stimulation was similar in humans (21%) and pigs (17%) (Figure 2.1D), which was on average 9-fold higher than in rabbits and sheep (both 2%) (p<0.001) and 2 to 3-fold higher than in rats (7%) (p=0.017).

Thrombin stimulation did not alter the ML in any species (Figure 2.1D).

**4.1.2. Endogenous thrombin potential (ETP)**

The median area under the curve (AUC) of thrombin generation in humans (4235 nM·min) and sheep (4092 nM·min) was 25% higher than in rats (3075 nM·min; p=0.042) and 50% higher than in pigs (2043 nM·min; p=0.019). The AUC in rabbits was higher than in humans and other species (6295 nM·min; p=0.02) (Figure 2.3).

The lag phase of thrombin generation (from addition of tissue factor until first burst of thrombin) was more than 90% higher in humans (12 min) than in other species (p<0.05) (Figure 2.3).

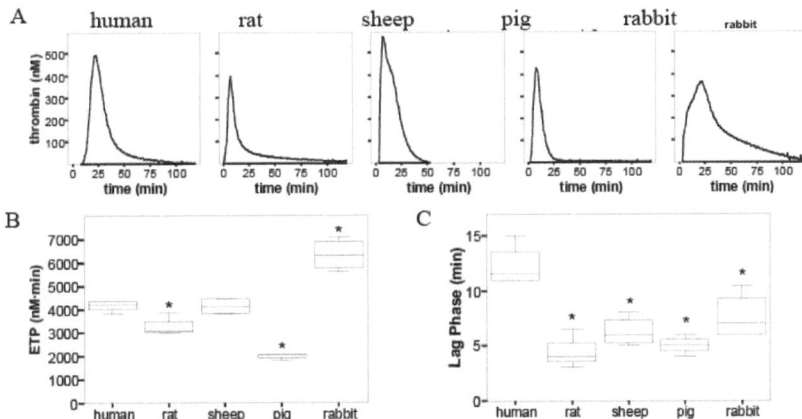

**Figure 2.3.** Endogenous thrombin generation in different species. **A)** Averaged curves of thrombin generation over time; **B)** Endogenous thrombin potential (ETP); **C)** Lag Phase of thrombin generation; *p<0.05 compared to human.

*Results*

### 4.1.3. Coagulation parameters at baseline

The fibrinogen levels in all species were in the normal range of human (180-390 mg/dl) (Figure 2.4). The median activated partial thromboplastin time (APTT) was on average >50% longer in rabbits (76s) than in other species (p=0.005). The median platelet counts (PLT) in rats (1180 x $10^9$/L), sheep (742 x $10^9$/L) and pigs (430 x $10^9$/L) were 6, 4 and 2 fold higher than in humans (187 x $10^9$/L) (p<0.001), respectively. In humans and rabbits, the platelet counts (PLT) were in the same range (160-330 x $10^9$/L). The median values of prothrombin time (PT) in humans (21s) and rabbits (20s) were 2-fold lower than in sheep (40s) (p<0.001) (Figure 2.4). The prothrombin time (PT) in rats (24s) and pigs (23s) was slightly longer than in humans (p<0.05).

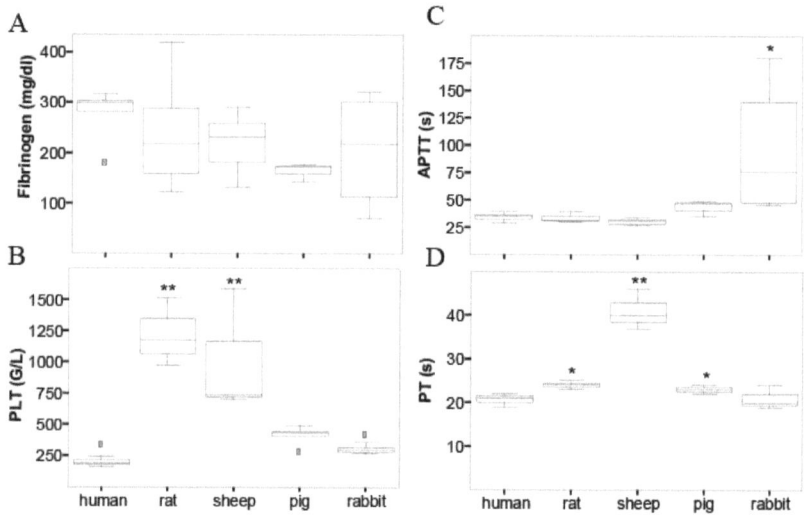

**Figure 2.4.** Comparison of coagulation parameters in different species. **A)** Fibrinogen **B)** Activated partial thromboplastin time (APTT); **C)** Platelets (PLT); **D)** Prothrombin time (PT). *p<0.05, **p<0.001 compared to human.

*Results*

# 4.2. STUDY II: A rat model of thrombin – induced consumption coagulopathy

### 4.2.1. DOSE ESCALATION

Six doses of thrombin were evaluated in a dose escalation study in 18 rats (n=3 per dose) and three rats served as a control group. The total minimal dose was 0.5 U/kg/min and the maximal dose was 0.9 U/kg/min (Table 3.1).

| Thrombin Dose (U) Cumulative U/kg | U/kg/min | Clinical symptoms/ organ pathology during autopsy | Organ histology | Lethal Outcome |
|---|---|---|---|---|
| 0 | 0 | Without pathological findings | Without pathological findings | 0/3 |
| 15 | 0.05 | Without pathological findings | Without pathological findings | 0/8 |
| 30 | 0.1 | Subcutaneous haemorrhage, intramural bladder haematoma, macrohematuria | Without pathological findings | 0/3 |
| 45 | 0.15 | Intramural intestinal haematoma, macrohematuria, liver haemorrhage, intraperitoneal bleeding | Liver oedema n=1 | 1/3 (2.5h after start of infusion) |
| 90 | 0.3 | Macrohematuria, intraperitoneal bleeding, liver haemorrhage, lung haemorrhage | Liver oedema n=1 Alveolar haemorrhage n=1 | 1/3 (4h after start of infusion) |
| 180 | 0.6 | Macrohematuria, subcutaneous haemorrhage | Without pathological findings | 0/3 |
| 270 | 0.9 | Macrohematuria, intraperitoneal bleeding, bleeding from the insertion site of the intravenous cannula, lung haemorrhage | Perivascular lung oedema n=1 Alveolar haemorrhage n=1 | 2/3 (2.5h and 4h after start of infusion) |

**Table 3.1.** Clinical symptoms, survival, macroscopic organ pathology and organ histology in the dose escalation and verification studies.

#### *4.2.1.1. Laboratory parameters*

Intravenous infusion of thrombin at doses of 0.05-0.6 U/kg/min did not significantly alter platelet counts or fibrinogen levels (Figure 3.1A and 3.1B). Thrombin infusion at a dose of 0.9 IU/kg/min decreased platelet count by 70% compared to the control group (median 230 vs. 752 x $10^9$/L; p=0.041; Figure 3.1A).

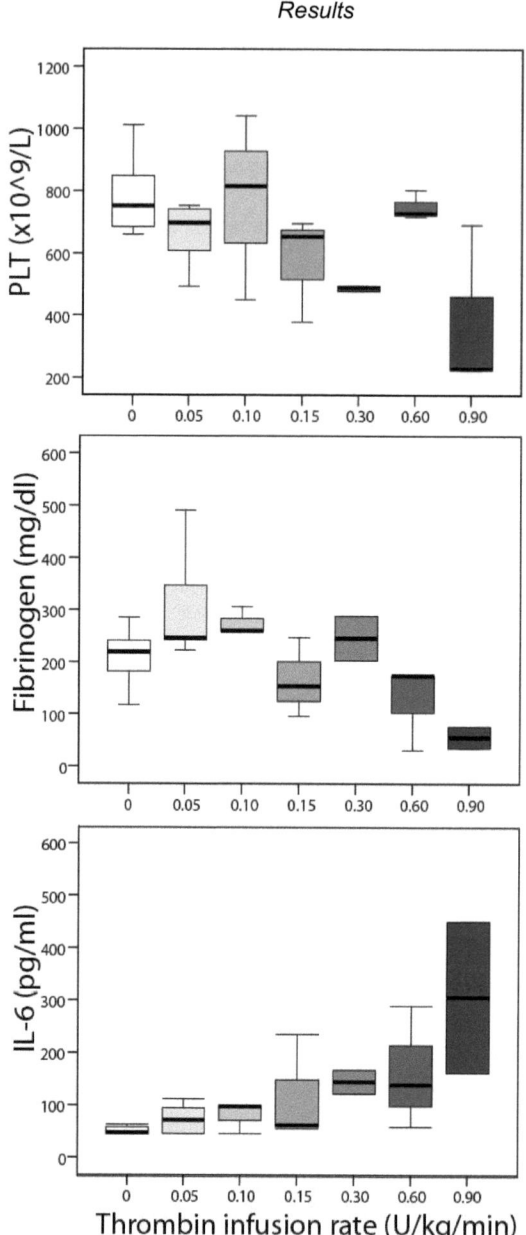

**Figure 3.1. A)** Platelet counts (PLT), **B)** fibrinogen levels and **C)** interleukin-6 levels (IL-6) immediately after the end of thrombin infusion in the dose escalation study.

*Results*

In accordance, infusion of 0.9 IU/kg/min of thrombin decreased fibrinogen by 75% compared to the control group (56mg/dl vs. 220mg/dl; p=0.046; Figure 3.1B). Although great variability in response to thrombin was observed, there was a trend toward a dose-dependent effect of thrombin on platelet count and fibrinogen level (Figure 3.1A and 3.1B). Thrombin infusion of up to 0.1 IU/kg/min did not alter the activated partial thromboplastin time (aPTT; data not shown). Changes in aPTT became significant after infusion of $\geq$0.15 U/kg/min thrombin (roughly 2- fold increase; 39s; p=0.032) and the majority of animals receiving $\geq$0.3 U/kg/min of thrombin displayed a maximal aPTT prolongation (>180s; p<001; data not shown). Doses $\geq$0.6 U/kg/min were needed to prolong the prothrombin time (1.8 -fold prolongation; 52s vs. 30s; p=0.014; data not shown). Thrombin infusion did not influence other laboratory parameters of coagulation (D-Dimer, thrombin time), haematology (white blood cell counts and red blood cell counts) or chemistry (alanine amino transferase (ALT), aspartate amino transferase (AST), lactate dehydrogenase (LDH), creatinine, blood urea nitrogen (BUN), glucose, lactate or pH; data not shown).

*4.2.1.2. Inflammation parameters*

Intravenous infusion of thrombin increased levels of IL-6 dose-dependently (Figure 3.1C). Administration of thrombin at doses of 0.3 and 0.6 IU/kg/min increased IL-6 levels 3-fold compared to the control group (139pg/ml, p=0.031; 144pg/ml, p=0.037 vs. 47pg/ml, respectively; Figure 3.1C). The level of IL-6 was 6.5-fold higher after infusion of a cumulative dose of 0.9 U/kg/min compared to the control group (306pg/ml, p=0.031; Figure 3.1C). In contrast, thrombin infusion did not significantly alter other markers of inflammation (TNF-alfa: <18.4pg/ml in the control group vs. <18.4pg/ml after thrombin infusion in all animals except two: 36.1pg/ml and 77pg/ml, p>0.05; MCP-1: 7.2µg/ml in the control group vs. 4.9-8.9µg/ml after thrombin infusion, p>0.05; IL-10: 20.2pg/ml in the control group vs. 10-57pg/ml after thrombin infusion, p>0.05; data not shown).

*4.2.1.3. Association between thrombin dose, platelet count, fibrinogen level and IL-6 level*

Thrombin doses correlated moderately with platelet counts and fibrinogen levels (R=-0.4; R=-0.58, p<0.005). In contrast, a good correlation was observed between thrombin doses and IL-6 levels (R=0.7; p<0.001).

*Results*

### *4.2.1.4. Symptoms of DIC and survival*

Thrombin infusion was lethal in four cases (Table 1). Death of animals was dose dependent and occurred at doses ≥0.15 IU/kg/min (4/12, 30%). Thrombin infusion caused bleedings but not thromboembolic events. Bleeding complications were observed at the earliest four hours after start of thrombin infusion. Thrombin at doses of ≥0.1 IU/kg/min caused macrohematuria, intramural bladder haematoma and subcutaneous bleeding (Table 3.1). Autopsy showed intraperitoneal bleeding, liver haemorrhage, lung haemorrhage, lung oedema and intramural intestinal haematoma at doses ≥0.15 IU/kg/min (Table 3.1; Figure 3.2). Thrombin infusion at doses of 0.9 IU/kg/min also produced bleeding from an insertion site of an intravenous cannula (Table 3.1). Anal temperature did not rise during thrombin infusion.

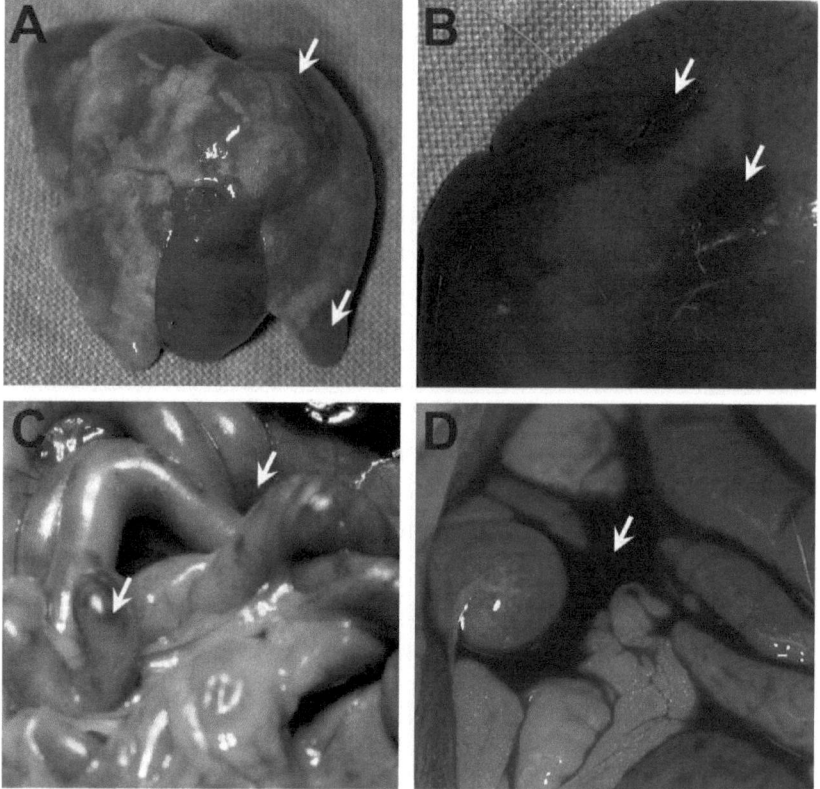

**Figure 3.2.** Organ pathology (macroscopic) after thrombin infusion in the dose escalation study: **A)** lung haemorrhage, **B)** liver haemorrhage **C)** intramural intestinal haematoma **D)** intraperitoneal bleeding. White arrows represent pathologic changes. Organs were extracted from animals immediately after the end of thrombin infusion.

*Results*

Histological examination showed alveolar haemorrhage in two rats (doses: 0.3 and 0.9 IU/kg/min; Figure 3.3), lung oedema (perivascular) in one rat (dose: 0.9 IU/kg/min; Figure 3.3) and liver oedema in two animals (doses: 0.15 and 0.3 IU/kg/min; Figure 3.3; hematoxylin and eosin stain). There was no evidence for intravascular thrombus formation at any thrombin dose (Masson trichrome stain; data not shown).

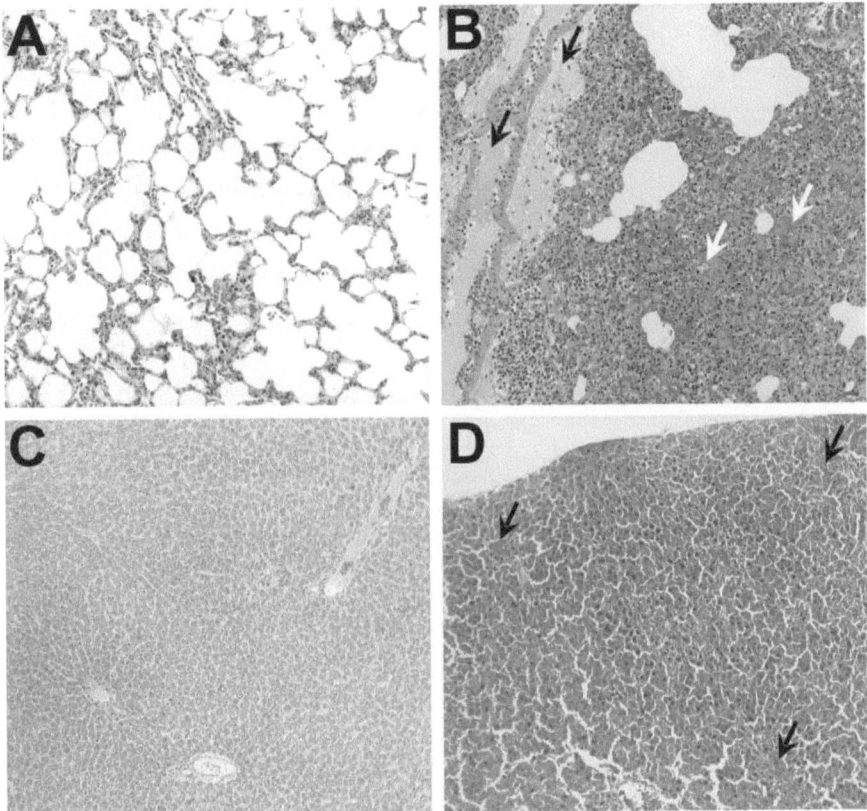

**Figure 3.3.** Organ pathology (microscopic) after thrombin infusion in the dose escalation study: **A)** control lung, **B)** lung in the treatment arm: alveolar haemorrhage (white arrow) and perivascular oedema (black arrow), **C)** control liver, **D)** liver in the treatment arm: oedema (black arrow); magnification 100x, hematoxylin and eosin stain. Organs were extracted from animals immediately after the end of thrombin infusion.

*Results*

*4.2.1.5. Estimates of safety and tolerability*

The "no observed adverse effect level" (*NOAEL*) of thrombin was 0.05 U/kg/min. The "lowest observed adverse effect level" (*LOAEL*) was 0.1 U/kg/min (Table 3.1).

*4.2.1.6. Association between platelet count, fibrinogen level, bleeding events and survival*

The median platelet count was 3.3- fold higher in animals, that survived (median 760 x $10^9$/L) compared to those, that died (230 x $10^9$/L; p=0.005; Figure 3.4A). Similarly, the median fibrinogen level was 3.2- fold higher in surviving rats compared to deceased animals (243mg/dl vs. 76mg/dl; p=0.011; Figure 3.4B). In accordance, platelet count and fibrinogen level were 1.5- and 1.4- fold higher in rats without any bleeding complications compared with those with bleeding events, (platelet count: 731 x $10^9$/L vs. 496 x $10^9$/L; p=0.022; Figure 3.4C; fibrinogen level: 243mg/dl vs. 174mg/dl; p=0.025; Figure 3.4D).

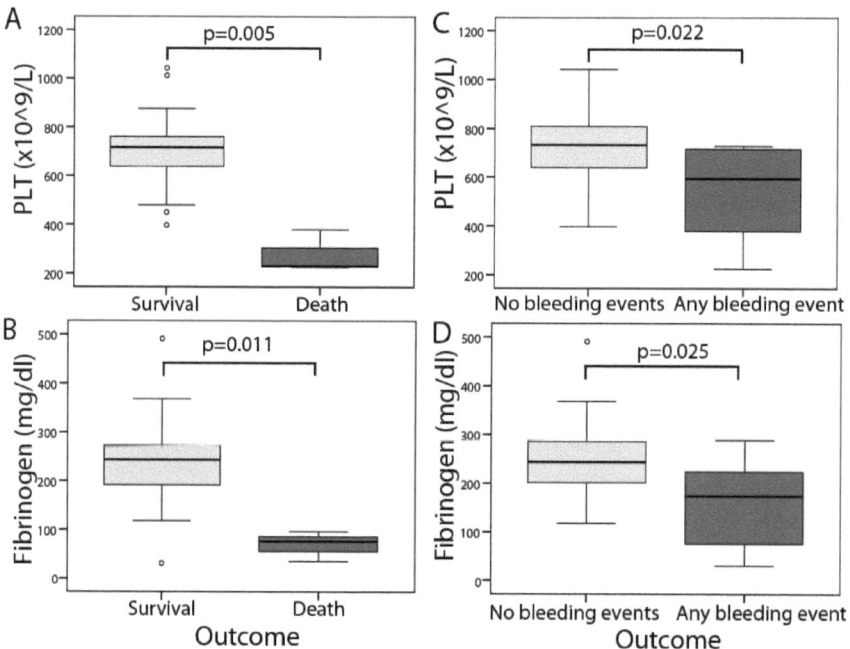

**Figure 3.4.** Association between levels of laboratory parameters and clinical outcome in the dose escalation study. **A)** platelet count (PLT) and survival, **B)** fibrinogen level and survival **C)** platelet count (PLT) and bleeding events, **D)** fibrinogen level and bleeding events. Blood was taken immediately after the end of thrombin infusion. In animals, which did not survive the values are reported for a time point prior to death.

*Results*

There was no difference in baseline values between rats, which survived vs. rats, which died or rats with bleedings vs. rats without bleedings (platelets: $1181 \times 10^9$/L vs. $1234 \times 10^9$/L, p>0.05; fibrinogen: 288 mg/dl vs. 312 mg/dl, p>0.05). No other measured parameters correlated with bleedings or survival. Interestingly, thrombocytopenia was strongly associated with bleeds (all animals, which developed bleeding complications had platelet counts under the normal range of $800 \times 10^9$/L), whereas a weaker effect was observed for fibrinogen depletion (50% of animals suffering from bleeds had fibrinogen levels under the normal range of 180 mg/dl).

## 4.2.2. DOSE VERIFICATION

To verify the safety and tolerability of infused thrombin at the "no observed adverse effect level" (NOAEL), five additional animals received cumulative thrombin doses of 0.05 IU/kg/min. Two animals were sacrificed immediately after the end of thrombin infusion and three animals were observed for 24 hours and subsequently sacrificed. Thrombin at this dose did not impair animal's behaviour and did not affect levels of laboratory parameters. There was no difference in laboratory parameters at time points 5h and 24h. Moreover, all animals survived and no pathological findings were found in autopsy or organ histology.

## 4.2.3. LEPIRUDIN/PLACEBO

The platelet counts in animals receiving simultaneously thrombin and lepirudin were 24% higher compared to the control group receiving thrombin/placebo ($827 \times 10^9$/L vs. $668 \times 10^9$/L; p=0.01; Figure 3.5A). In contrast, there was no difference in the fibrinogen levels between both study groups (223mg/dl vs. 228mg/dl; p=0.688; Figure 3.5B). This might be explained by the fact that a thrombin dose of 0.3 IU/kg/min also did not alter the fibrinogen level in the dose escalation study. Therefore, higher concentrations of thrombin might be required for the evaluation of the potentially protective effect of lepirudin on fibrinogen level.

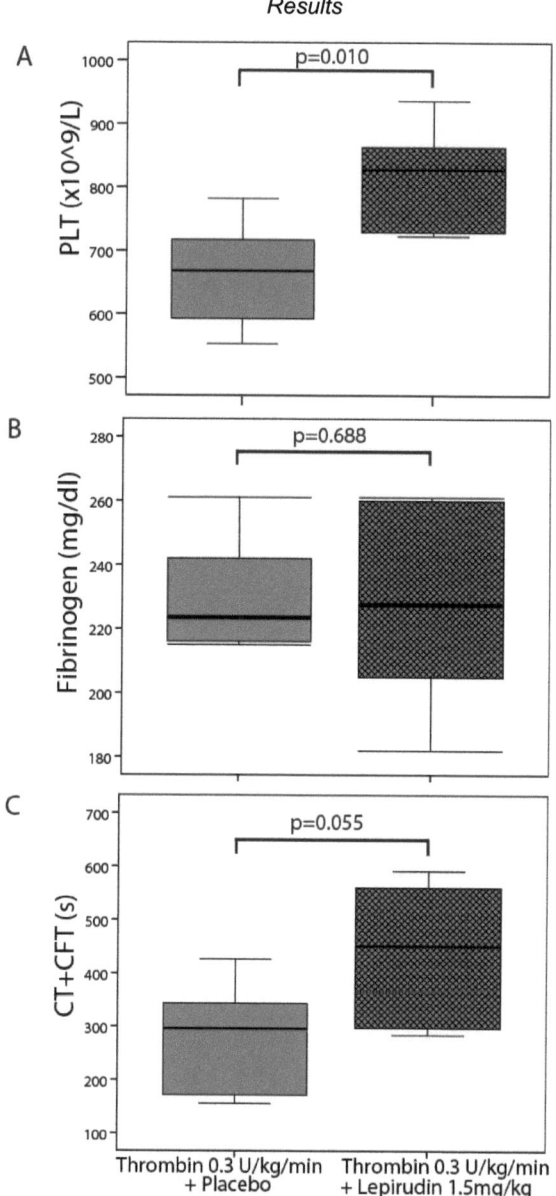

**Figure 3.5.** Effects of lepirudin vs. placebo on **A)** platelet counts (PLT), **B)** fibrinogen levels and **C)** sum of clotting time and clot formation time (CT+CFT) in animals receiving thrombin (0.3 U/kg/min). Blood was taken immediately after the end of thrombin infusion.

*Results*

Anticoagulant properties of lepirudin were reflected by a 52% prolongation in the clotting time and clot formation time, which represent activation and dynamics of clot formation (451s vs. 296s; p=0.055; Figure 3.5C).

Three animals receiving placebo + thrombin developed bleedings (two intraperitoneal and one macrohaematuria) and one rat receiving lepirudin suffered from an intraperitoneal bleeding (p=0.221). There were no lethal outcomes.

*Results*

## 4.3. STUDY III: An ovine model of thrombin – induced consumption coagulopathy

### 4.3.1. DOSE ESCALATION

In the dose escalation study eleven doses of thrombin were evaluated. In three control experiments sheep received physiologic saline solution. The total minimal cumulative dose was 0.13 IU/kg (0.0004 IU/kg/min) and the maximal dose was 125 IU/kg (0.42 IU/kg/min; Table 4.1; Figure 4.1).

| Cumulative thrombin dose (IU/kg) | Infusion rate (IU/kg/min) | Clinical symptoms of DIC | Laboratory confirmation of DIC | Lethal Outcome |
|---|---|---|---|---|
| 0 | 0 | None | None | 0/6 |
| 0.13 | 0.0004 | None | None | 0/1 |
| 0.25 | 0.0008 | None | None | 0/1 |
| 0.50 | 0.0016 | None | None | 0/2 |
| 1 | 0.0033 | None | None | 0/2 |
| 2 | 0.0067 | None | None | 0/1 |
| 4 | 0.0133 | None | None | 0/1 |
| 8 | 0.0267 | None | None | 0/1 |
| 13 | 0.0433 | None | None | 0/1 |
| 32 | 0.1067 | None | Fibrinogen↓ | 0/1 |
| 64 | 0.2133 | None | Fibrinogen↓, TT↑ | 0/1 |
| 125 | 0.4166 | None * | Fibrinogen↓, PLT↓, TT↑, aPTT↑ | 0/5 |

**Table 4.1.** Clinical symptoms, survival, macroscopic organ pathology and organ histology in the dose escalation and verification studies. * findings in histology: lung haemorrhage and pulmonary oedema. PLT=platelets; TT=thrombin time; aPTT=activated partial thromboplastin time.

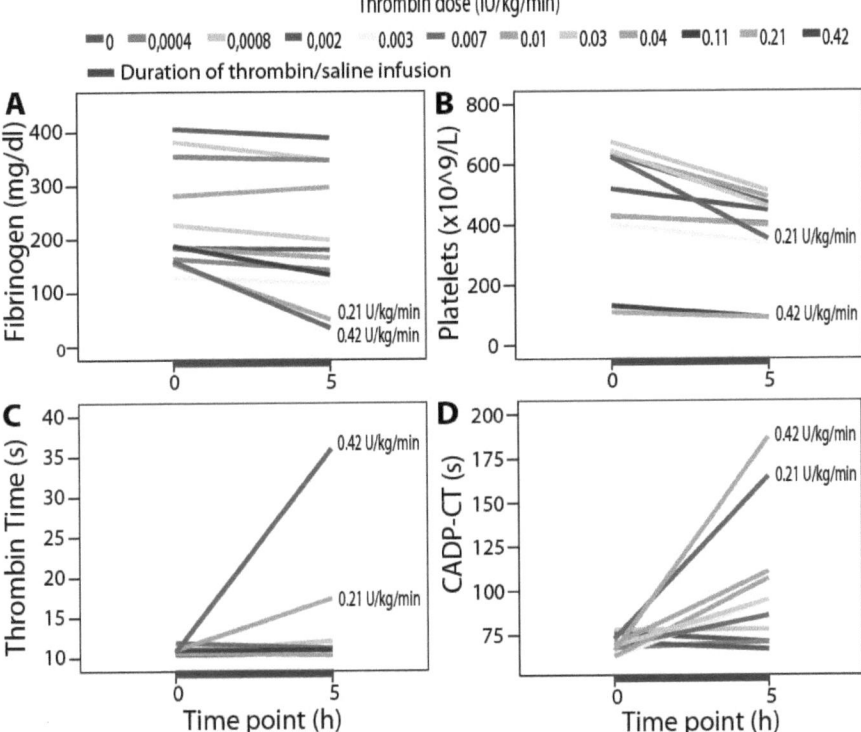

**Figure 4.1.** Effects of different thrombin doses on **A)** fibrinogen levels, **B)** platelet counts, **C)** thrombin time, and **D)** collagen/adenosine diphosphate induced closure time (CADP-CT) at baseline and at 5 hours (immediately after the end of thrombin infusion) in the dose escalation study.

*4.3.1.1. Coagulation parameters*

Intravenous infusion of thrombin at doses of 0.004-0.1 IU/kg/min did not significantly alter any of the laboratory parameters. Thrombin doses of 0.21-0.42 IU/kg/min decreased fibrinogen levels, prolonged the thrombin time and collagen/adenosine diphosphate closure time (Figure 4.1A-D). A decrease in platelet counts or prolongation of the thrombin time (TT) were first observed after infusion of 0.42 IU/kg/min of thrombin (Figure 4.1B). A thrombin dose of 0.42 IU/kg/min was chosen for the dose verification study due to a fibrinogen and platelet effect. Infusion of thrombin did not significantly alter D-Dimer likely due to a lack of cross reactivity in the assay used.

The thrombin dose correlated moderately with the fibrinogen level (R=-0.52; p=0.012). In contrast, good correlation was noted for the thrombin dose and the thrombin time (R=0.87; p<0.001).

*Results*

The applied thrombin doses did not influence blood counts or any of the chemistry parameters (alanine amino transferase, aspartate amino transferase, lactate dehydrogenase, creatinine, blood urea nitrogen, glucose, lactate or pH).

*4.3.1.2. Estimates of safety and tolerability*

Infusion of thrombin neither caused clinical symptoms of DIC nor had lethal effects. The no observed adverse effect level (*NOAEL*) was 0.04 IU/kg/min, the lowest observed adverse effect level (*LOAEL*) was 0.1 IU/kg/min (Table 4.1).

**4.3.2. DOSE VERIFICATION**

The maximal thrombin dose (0.42 IU/kg/min) was verified in three additional animals in a cross over design (thrombin vs. control: 0.9% saline solution) with a wash out period of one week.

*4.3.2.1. Coagulation parameters*

Thrombin decreased fibrinogen levels by 75-87% at 5 hours (mean 40-45mg/dl) as compared to baseline (158mg/dl; p<0.01) or to the control group (178mg/dl; p<0.001; Figure 4.2A). Interestingly, fibrinogen levels did not recover to baseline during the whole observation period (Figure 4.2A). The nadir in platelet counts (36%) was observed at 5 hours (584 vs. 373 x $10^9$/L; p=0.006; Figure 4.2B). Thrombin prolonged the thrombin time by 70% at 5 hours (11s vs. 36s; p=0.012; Figure 4.2C) with return of values to baseline at 48 hours. The 32% prolongation of aPTT at 5 hours did not reach statistical significance in the low sample size (Figure 4.2D).

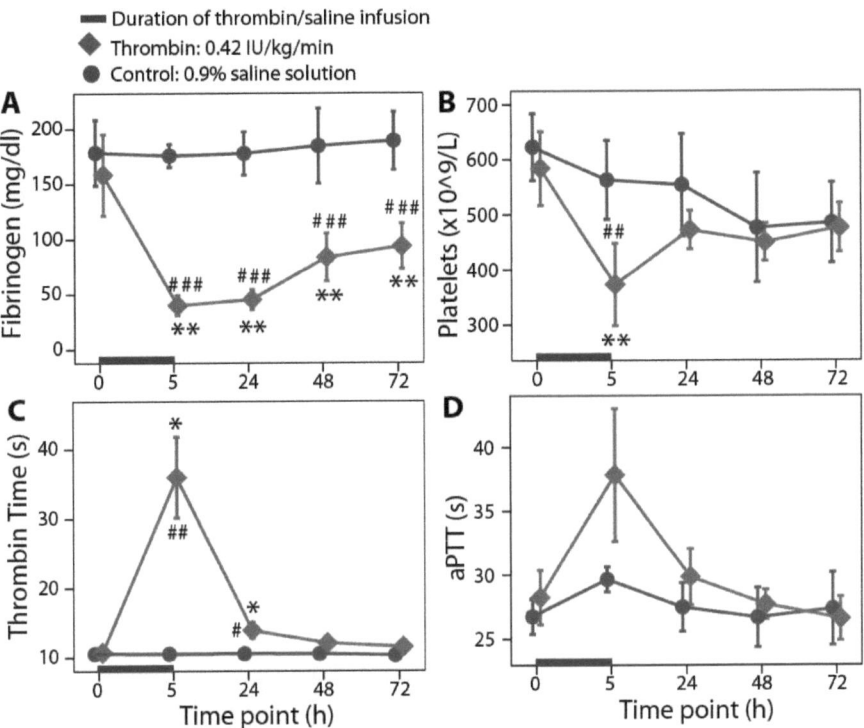

**Figure 4.2.** Thrombin effects (0.42IU/kg/min) on **A)** fibrinogen levels, **B)** platelet counts, **C)** thrombin time, and **D)** activated partial thromboplastin time (aPTT) at baseline (0 hours) and after the end of thrombin infusion (5-72 hours) in the dose verification study. * compared to baseline; # compared to the control group; * $p<0.05$; ** $p<0.01$; *** $p<0.005$; # $p<0.05$; ## $p<0.01$; ### $p<0.005$.

In order to define the time point at which thrombin starts to alter laboratory parameters during its infusion, additional blood samples were taken hourly in one animal (Figure 4.3). Thrombin decreased fibrinogen levels already after 1 hour with a maximal effect at 3 to 5 hours (Figure 4.3A). The nadir in platelet counts was observed already at 1 hour (figure 4.3B). In contrast, thrombin prolonged the thrombin time and the aPTT maximally at 5 hours (Figure 4.3C and 4.3D).

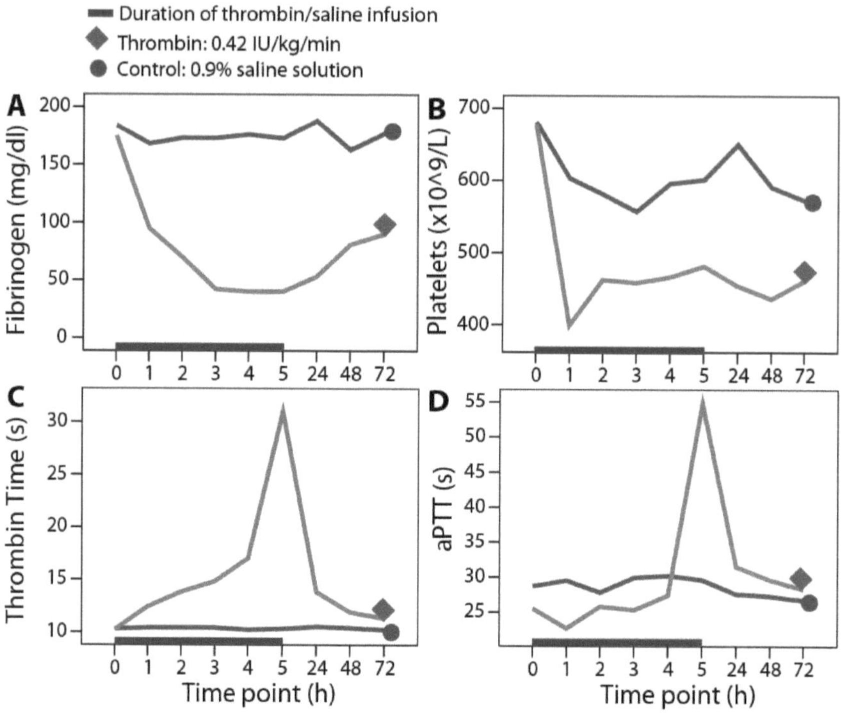

*Results*

**Figure 4.3.** Time dependence of the thrombin effects on **A)** fibrinogen levels, **B)** platelet counts, **C)** thrombin time, and **D)** activated partial thromboplastin time (aPTT) during (at 1,2,3,4 hours) and after the end of thrombin infusion (5-72 hours) in the dose verification study.

Thrombin increased the activity of coagulation factors FV by 27% (p=0.045; Figure 4.4A) and that of FX by 40% (p=0.012; Figure 4.4C) maximally at 5 hours. Thrombin did not affect FX assay sensitivity, which was demonstrated in an additional experiment, where FX deficient plasma was incubated with thrombin *in vitro* (data not shown). In contrast, thrombin decreased the activity of the FVIII by 53% (p=0.001; Figure 4.4B) and the FXIII by 25% (p=0.012; Figure 4.4D). Other coagulation factors were not affected by thrombin infusion (data not shown).

Results

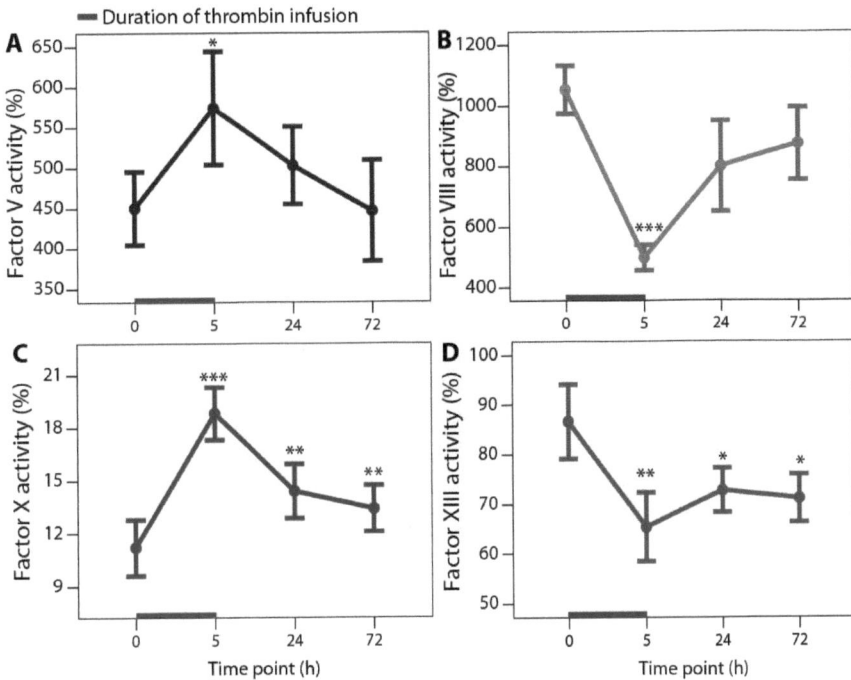

**Figure 4.4.** Thrombin effects (0.42IU/kg/min) on levels of coagulation factors **A)** Va, **B)** VIIIa, **C)** Xa and **D)** XIIIa in animals receiving 125IU/kg thrombin at baseline (0 hours) and after the end of thrombin infusion (5-72 hours) in the dose verification study. * $p<0.05$; ** $p<0.01$; *** $p<0.005$.

### 4.3.2.2. Proteomics and mass spectrometry analysis

Thrombin decreased the concentration of fibrinogen alpha chain (Figure 4.5B: green spots at 65 kD - oval 1; identification in Table 4.2) and fibrinogen beta chain (Figure 4.5B: green spots at 60 kD - oval 2; identification in Table 4.2) compared to baseline and to the control (Figure 4.5C). Fibrinogen was reduced by a factor of 2 to 5 at time points 5-72 hours. The decrease was slightly higher for the fibrinogen beta chain. In contrast, thrombin elevated a breakdown product of the fibrinogen beta chain 3 to 5 -fold at 5 hours (Figure 4.5B: red spots at 41 kD - oval 3; identification in Table 4.2). This breakdown product of the fibrinogen beta chain was not detectable at any later time point. No changes in other plasma proteins were detected in the proteomic analysis.

*Results*

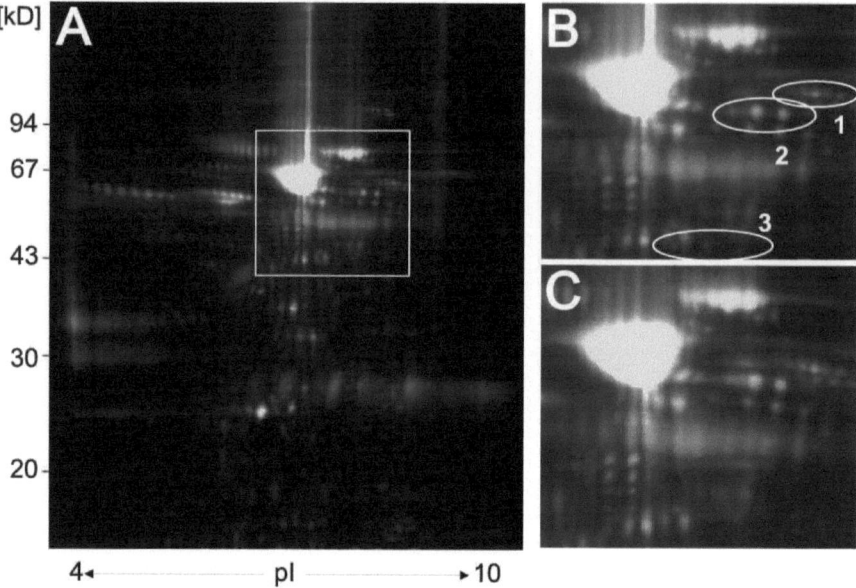

**Figure 4.5.** Proteomic analysis: 2D-DIGE of sheep plasma. Figure **A)** complete gel image from one of the animals, which received thrombin infusion (0.42IU/kg/min); overlay of two samples from time course experiment; sample 1) before treatment, colour coding green; sample 2) time point 5h, colour coding red; overlap of samples 1) and 2) colour coding yellow (corresponding to proteins with similar concentration pre and post thrombin infusion). The white square indicates the area displayed in the close-ups B (treated animal) and C (control animal). Figure **B)** represents samples from animal receiving thrombin infusion. The white ellipses marking the green spots represent proteins down-regulated at 5h: **1)** fibrinogen alpha chains and **2)** fibrinogen beta chains. **3)** The white ellipse marking the red spots represents a breakdown product of fibrinogen beta chain, which is up-regulated at 5h. Figure **C)** represents the respective samples of a control animal.

| Spot chain in Figure 5B | Peptides | Protein |
|---|---|---|
| 1 | K.QLEQVIAINLLPSR.D | Fibrinogen chain A (P02672) |
| 2 | K.LESDVSTQMEYCR.T R.TMTIHNSMFFSTYDR.D K.EDGGGWWYNR.C | Fibrinogen chain B (P02676) |
| 3 | K.IQKLESDVSTQMEYCR.T K.EDGGGWWYNR.C R.QDGSVDFGR.K K.GGWTVIQNR.Q | Fibrinogen chain B (P02676) – break down products |

**Table 4.2.** Tryptic peptides identified by the mass spectrometry analysis of the three spot chains marked in Figure 4.5B. The identification was assumed based on the similarity of the peptides to the respective bovine homologues (data for sheep are not available) and their position on the gel being similar to the ones described for fibrinogen single chains of other species [133].

## 4.3.2.3. Thromboelastometry

Thrombin infusion significantly altered clot formation, which was reflected in a 7-fold prolongation of clotting time and clot formation time (CT+CFT) at 5 hours (726s vs. 4999s; p=0.019; Figure 4.6A) with a return to the baseline at 24 hours. Thrombin profoundly decreased clot firmness (MCF; 65mm vs. 23mm; p<0.001; Figure 4.6B) and the alpha angle at 5 hours (54° vs. 9°; p<0.001; 4.6C). Interestingly, MCF and alpha angle did not return to baseline values during the study period (p<0.05; Figures 4.6B and 4.6C); both parameters correlated with fibrinogen levels at each time point (R=0.8-0.9; p<0.001).

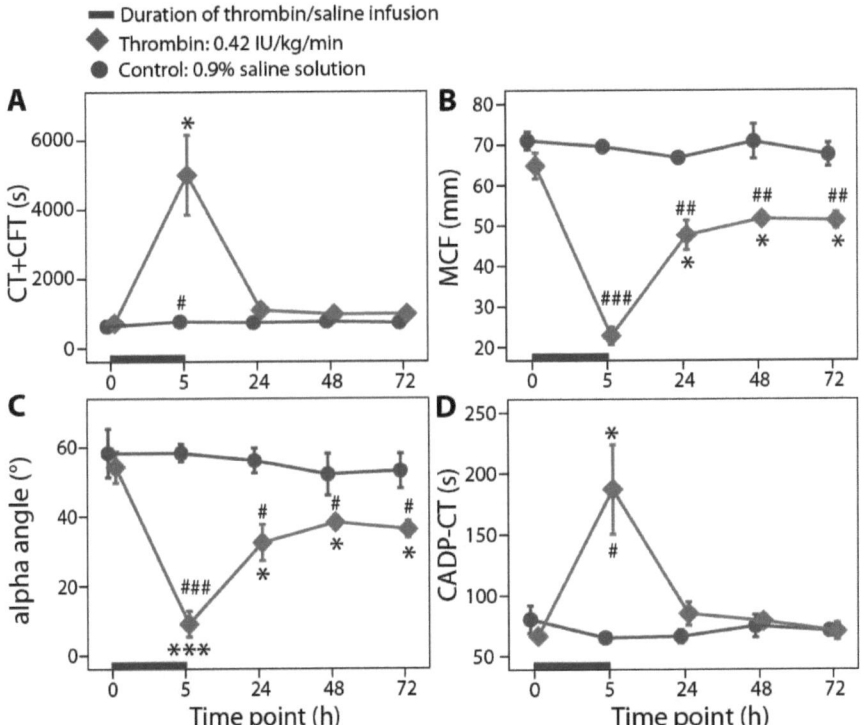

**Figure 4.6.** Thrombin effects (0.42IU/kg/min) on thromboelastography parameters: **A)** the sum of clotting time and clot formation time (CT+CFT), **B)** maximal clot firmness (MCF) and **C)** alpha angle. **D)** Thrombin effects on collagen/adenosine diphosphate induced closure time (CADP-CT) in the PFA -100 at baseline (0 hours) and after the end of thrombin infusion (5-72 hours) in the dose verification study.

*4.3.2.4. Platelet Function*

Thrombin did not impair the ADP-induced platelet aggregation. Thrombin decreased collagen- induced platelet aggregation at 5 hours (8U vs. 1.2U; p=0.12; data not shown), but ovine platelets were not very sensitive to the collagen used. Similarly, ovine platelets were not sensitive to TRAP. Thrombin affected shear-dependent platelet function, which was reflected in a 3- fold prolongation of the collagen/adenosine diphosphate closure time at 5 hours (CADP-CT; 66s vs. 187s; p=0.031; Figure 4.6D). This is in accordance with a 24% reduction in the von Willebrand factor-ristocetin cofactor activity (vWF:RICO) at 5 hours (p<0.001; Figure 7A).

*4.3.2.5. Thrombin generation assay*

Of note, thrombin infusion decreased the capacity of blood to generate thrombin. The maximal effect was observed at 5 hours (Figure 4.7B). The drop in generated thrombin persisted during the whole study period (Figure 4.7B), which is in accordance with the fibrinogen course (Figure 4.2A).

*Results*

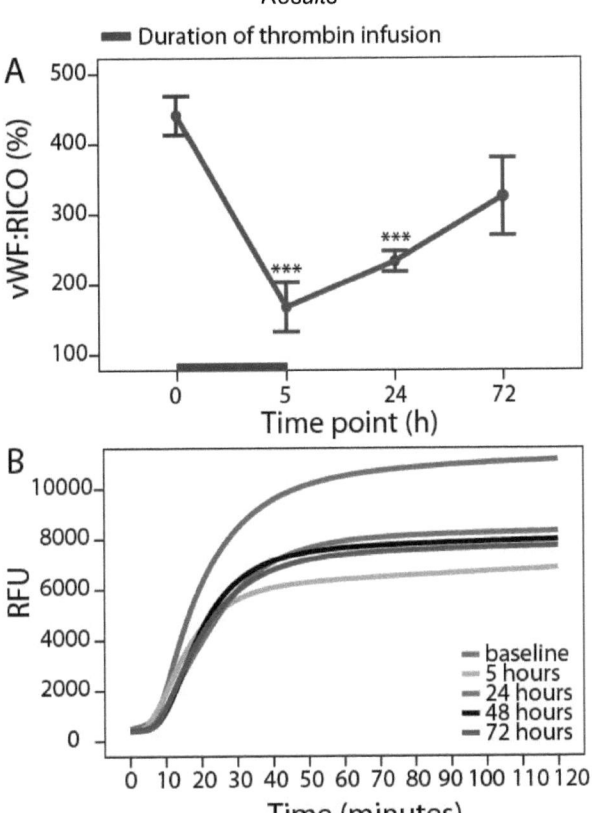

**Figure 4.7.** Thrombin effects on **A)** von Willebrand factor – ristocetin cofactor activity (vWF:RICO) and **B)** relative fluorescence intensity (RFU) in the thrombin generation assay (TGA) in animals receiving 0.42IU/kg/min thrombin at baseline (0 hours) and after the end of thrombin infusion (5-72 hours) in the dose verification study. *** $p<0.005$.

### *4.3.2.6. Symptoms of DIC, Survival and Organ Pathology*

Thrombin did not cause clinical symptoms of DIC, had no lethal effects and did not impair animal behaviour. Nevertheless, autopsy showed lung haemorrhage in all animals receiving 0.42 IU/kg/min of thrombin (Figure 4.8B). This finding was confirmed in histological examination, which yielded alveolar haemorrhage and peri-vascular lung oedema in all animals (Figure 4.8D; hematoxylin and eosin stain). There was no evidence for intravascular thrombus formation (Masson trichrome stain) and no other organ pathology.

*Results*

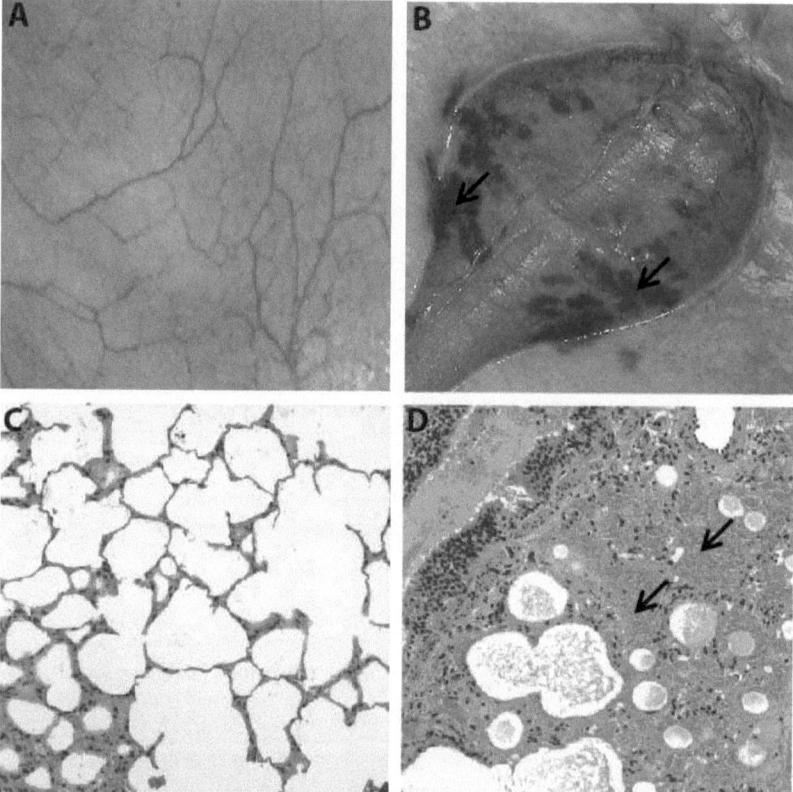

**Figure 4.8.** Organ pathology after thrombin infusion in the dose verification study (0.42IU/kg/min): **A)** control lung (macroscopic) **B)** lung haemorrhage after infusion of 125 IU of thrombin (macroscopic; arrow), **C)** control lung (haematoxylin and eosin stain) **D)** lung after infusion of 125 IU of thrombin (haematoxylin and eosin stain): alveolar haemorrhage (arrow). Organs were extracted from animals at day 8.

# 5. DISCUSSION
## 5.1 Interspecies differences in coagulation profile

Our data on species comparison of the coagulation profile are novel because to our knowledge there are no published data on interspecies differences in the clot formation and subsequent lysis.

In humans and sheep, a 100-fold lower dose of thrombin (0.002 IU) was required to shorten the clotting time (CT) as compared to rats, pigs and rabbits (0.2 IU) (Figure 2.1A). Moreover, thrombin doses higher than 0.2 IU did not have a significant additional effect on the clotting time in any species. The highest dose of thrombin was chosen on the basis of a previous report, which showed shortening in the clotting time after incubation of human and pig blood with 1 IU of thrombin [134]. These data are novel and provide more complete understanding of interspecies differences in the thrombin effects on coagulation *in vitro*, which add to previously reported species differences of thrombin effects on platelet function [135-137].

Similar to the shortening of CT by thrombin, a thrombin dose >0.06 IU caused a decrease in the maximum clot firmness (MCF) in humans and rabbits (Figure 2.1C). A likely explanation for this could be that high doses of thrombin may lead to platelet aggregation and thereby decrease platelet counts, which results in a reduction of MCF. In contrast to humans and rabbits, thrombin did not cause changes in the MCF in pigs, rats and sheep, which may be due to higher doses of thrombin required. This explanation is supported by other investigators [135-137].

Moreover, this study provides evidence that thrombin did not cause changes in the maximal lysis (ML) in any species. Therefore, thrombin had no anti/fibrinolytic properties in this *in vitro* assay. A possible explanation of why thrombin did not alter fibrinolysis in our experiment might be an impaired activity of the thrombin-activable fibrinolysis inhibitor (TAFI) *in vitro*. The physiologic activator of TAFI is the thrombin-thrombomodulin complex [138]. Thrombomodulin is a transmembrane protein expressed in endothelial cells. The extracellular region of thrombomodulin is digested by proteases into diverse-sized fragments collectively called soluble thrombomodulin [139]. It has been reported that TAFI can be activated *in vitro* in the presence of either membrane-bound thrombomodulin or recombinant soluble thrombomodulin [140]. In the NATEM test, the endothelial transmembrane receptor thrombomodulin was not present. Therefore, the concentration of plasma soluble thrombomodulin in the blood is conceivably too low for activation of TAFI.

*Discussion*

The data obtained in this study indicate that sheep could be a suitable species for coagulation studies. First, humans and sheep have very similar dynamics of clot formation. The clotting times (CT) and the clot formation times (CFT), which represent the dynamics of clot formation were in the same range with or without thrombin stimulation in both species (Figure 2.1). In addition, thrombin shortened the clotting time (CT) with a similar half maximal effective concentration ($EC_{50}$) of 0.01 IU for humans and 0.02 IU for sheep (Figure 2.2). Second, humans and sheep had very similar AUC of the endogenous thrombin potential (ETP) (Figure 2.3). ETP is triggered by the addition of exogenous tissue factor and is a parameter for plasma-based hypercoagulability [141]. Third, activated partial thromboplastin time (aPTT) is used to measure the activity of factors of the so called intrinsic coagulation system. Comparable aPTT values in humans and sheep support the concept that there are no major differences in the intrinsic system between those two species (Figure 2.4).

These results thus lend further credence to studies on anticoagulant drugs in sheep including studies on heparin [142-145], warfarin [146] and gabexate mesilate [147]. Studies examining the efficacy of heparin in sheep have shown that heparin doses were directly applicable to humans [143]. However, it has been shown that the anticoagulant activities of heparins with different molecular weight differ between humans and sheep [148]. In particular, the efficacy of low molecular weight heparins was higher as compared to humans [148].

A comparison of the intrinsic and extrinsic coagulation system as well as the fibrinolytic system of five different species (human, sheep, pig, dog and rabbit) has shown that the coagulation system of humans exhibits similarities to that of sheep [145]. In contrast to the other species, which all have enhanced coagulation, the coagulation system of sheep was characterised by a slightly decreased activation of coagulation system as compared to humans [145]. Thus, the results of our study confirm this observation and support the concept that sheep could be the most suitable animal species for coagulation studies [145].

However, there were also differences between humans and sheep in our study. In the endogenous thrombin generation assay, the lag phase of thrombin generation, which represents the clotting time, was shorter in sheep than in humans (Figure 2.3). One possible explanation for this might be the different sensitivity of each species to the recombinant human tissue factor, which was the activator in the endogenous thrombin generation assay [149]. Apparently sheep blood seems to have higher sensitivity to the human tissue factor than human blood.

*Discussion*

In contrast to activated partial thromboplastin time (aPTT), sheep had longer prothrombin time (PT) values than humans. This is in agreement with another study [150]. Other publications reported shorter PT values than in our study (15-20s), however without direct comparison to humans [151,152]. This difference in study results may in part be explained by the assay used. We used a PT modified by Owen (Normotest), which is high sensitive to factor VII. As sheep are known to have decreased plasma levels of factor VII [145,152], this is likely explanation for differences in study results.

Similarly, differences between human and sheep in platelet reactivity to different agonists as well as differences in the activity of the von Willebrand factor have been previously described [153-155]. Nevertheless, sheep are widely used species for testing of artery grafts [147], synthetic devices [156] and extracorporeal circulation [144] due to the similarities between human and sheep in platelet adhesion to foreign surfaces [157].

A 100-fold higher dose of thrombin was required to cause a decrease in clotting time in rats as compared to humans (Figure 2.1A). This observation is supported by previous studies using different methods. Platelets of rats were at least 4-fold less responsive to thrombin when compared to human platelets when aggregometry was used [135,136]. Rats were 3-fold less responsive to thrombin than human platelets as measured by flow cytometry [137]. Also, anticoagulant and antiplatelet drug effects are different in rats and humans. A 40-fold higher dose of the potent inhibitor of factor Xa DX-9065a was required to inhibit thrombus formation in a rat thrombosis model as compared to humans [158]. In another study, prasugrel's active metabolite has been shown to inhibit platelet aggregation with a 3-fold higher $IC_{50}$ for rats as compared to humans [159]. Thus, these results indicate that pronounced species differences between humans and rats are a limitation for the usefulness of rats in the research on blood coagulation.

Humans and pigs had similar values of the maximum lysis of the clot (ML) (Figure 2.1D). Due to the similarities in the functional structure of coagulation proteins between humans and pigs [160], the usefulness of porcine plasmin for thrombolytic treatment in humans has been investigated [161]. In addition, a cross species comparison of the proteolytic activity of plasmin activated by the staphylokinase has shown that there are major similarities between humans and pigs [162]. However, an *in vitro* study has shown decreased sensitivity of porcine plasminogen to human tissue plasminogen activator [134]. Thus, our findings confirm the potential usefulness of pig as an experimental animal species for examining the fibrinolytic pathway [163-168]. Previous examples include studies examining the effects of plasminogen activators for prevention of the adult respiratory

## Discussion

distress syndrome [164], urokinase in disseminated intravascular coagulation model [165] and studies on tissue-type plasminogen activator [166,167].

Rabbits and humans had similar values of the maximum clot firmness (MCF) with and without thrombin stimulation (Figure 2.1C). The maximum clot firmness (MCF), which represents the clot strength and stability and describes platelet function, largely depends on platelet counts and fibrinogen [117,118,169]. Our study shows that humans and rabbits had similar platelet counts (PLT) and fibrinogen levels, which explain the similar MCF values. Thus, our results support the usefulness of rabbits as an animal species for examining platelets, which has been shown in previous studies [159,170-172]. A cross species comparison of the antiplatelet effect of prasugrel has shown most similar IC50 values between humans, rabbits and dogs, higher IC50 value for monkey and the highest for rats [159]. Moreover, it has been shown that the use of rabbits for studies examining platelet activation and aggregation *in vivo* in a model of arterial thrombosis is more advantageous as compared to other animals [171]. In addition, P2Y12 antagonists prevented arterial thrombosis in rabbits and suggested a reduction of thrombotic events in humans, which has been confirmed in clinical trials [173-175]. However, it has been shown that rabbit platelets do not contain plasminogen activator inhibitor-1 (PAI-1), which could be a limitation for usefulness of rabbits for studies on platelets [176].

### 5.2 Animal models of thrombin – induced consumption coagulopathy

Protracted intravenous infusion of thrombin over a period of five hours induced a haemorrhagic state in rats and sheep indicating that thrombin up to doses of 0.9IU/kg/min displays predominantly pro-hemorrhagic effects. In contrast to sheep where thrombin had no lethal effects, thrombin caused death in some rats, which correlated with the severity of changes in laboratory parameters of DIC.

Several groups have studied the effects of intravenous thrombin infusion in animals [65,66,68,71-74,77]. In most cases the objective was to establish a model to study thrombin-induced thromboembolism or thrombosis [73,86,95]. In most instances thrombin was infused into animals as a bolus or as an infusion which did not exceed one hour [77,99,177]. To our knowledge, thrombin infusion in animals over a period of at least two hours was studied only in four experiments [74,81,82,96]. Only two studies aimed to establish a model of thrombin-induced DIC [81,82]. The infusion rate of thrombin used in dogs (1.2U/kg/min; n=20) [82] and rabbits (1.6U/kg/min; n=35) [81] is similar to those used in our dose escalation study (0.9U/kg/min; n=3). Intravenous infusions of thrombin in rabbits initiated intravascular coagulation but did not result in deposition of fibrin [81]. Continuous thrombin infusion in

*Discussion*

dogs produced a progressive decrease in fibrinogen levels and thrombocytopenia without evidence of a thrombo-embolic state [82], which is in agreement with our results. The most probable cause for the thrombocytopenia is the agglutination of platelets due to activation via PAR1/4 receptors [28].

When thrombin was infused slowly at steady-state conditions, no intravascular clotting but bleedings occurred (Tables 3.1 and 4.1; Figures 3.2, 3.3 and 4.8), which indicates that without damage of endothelium or alterations in the vessel wall the fibrinolytic and anticoagulant properties of thrombin may overweigh. Interestingly, although the study in dogs reported prolongation in clotting times, bleeding events were not observed [82]. This difference with regard to bleedings between the study in dogs [82] and our study might be due to interspecies differences in the effects of thrombin [119]. An alternative explanation for this discrepancy could be the duration of thrombin infusion. As all bleeding complications were observed at the earliest four hours after start of thrombin infusion in our study, one can hypothesized that thrombin infusion in dogs for two hours [82] might have been too short to cause bleedings. Therefore, it might be possible that prolonged thrombin infusion over certain time period is essential for the occurrence of bleedings. This assumption could be strengthened by the observation that in critically ill patients with consumptive coagulopathy bleedings usually occur hours later than laboratory signs of coagulation activation [178,179].

In accordance with our results is a study in baboons, which has demonstrated that systemic infusion of thrombin at doses of 1-2U/kg/min reduced platelet and fibrin deposition on Dacron grafts in a protein C dependent manner [180]. Thus activation of protein C by thrombin may also have contributed to the antithrombotic effects of thrombin in this rat study e.g. by inactivation of plasminogen activator inhibitors (PAIs) [181]. Our study and the study in baboons [180] therefore indicate that thrombin at low concentrations is a much more antithrombotic than procoagulant factor, which is due to the activation of protein C.

Some rats developed intraperitoneal bleeding, lung- or liver oedema (Table 3.1, Figure 3.2 and 3.3), which might be explained by a thrombin- induced increase in endothelial permeability. Indeed, activation of PAR-1 receptors by thrombin is well-known to increase endothelial permeability secondary to disassembly of adherens junctions and actinomyosin contractility mechanism involving myosin light chain phosphorylation [182].

Interestingly, thrombin induced a moderate thrombocytopenia in sheep (36% drop in platelet count) only after infusion of the highest dose, which might indicate that human thrombin can not exert its full effect on ovine platelets [119]. This could be due to structural

*Discussion*

differences in proteinase- activated receptors (PAR1/4) between humans and sheep. In agreement with this hypothesis is that ovine platelets were insensitive to stimulation with thrombin receptor activating peptide (TRAP), which is an agonist on human PAR-1 receptor. Although interspecies differences in the structure and function of PAR receptors are well known [25-27], data on ovine platelet PAR receptors are to our knowledge lacking.

The decrease in fibrinogen levels in sheep was confirmed in a proteomic analysis showing a decrease of fibrinogen at all time points. A degradation product of the fibrinogen beta chain was detected at 5h, the time point of the lowest fibrinogen plasma level (Figure 4.2). Due to the rapid clearance of this breakdown product and no further thrombin infusion the respective spot chain was not detectable at a later time point.

Similar to changes in sheep, thrombin induced a decrease in platelet counts and fibrinogen in rats, whose severity was associated with bleeding complications and death (Figure 3.4). The direct thrombin inhibitor lepirudin prevented thrombin- induced thrombocytopenia (Figure 3.5A). This could be clinically useful because acquired thrombocytopenia is associated with worse clinical outcome [183].

Our data indicate that when the rate of thrombin infusion is carefully controlled doses up to 0.05 IU/kg/min can be given without causing any alterations in coagulation parameters (Table 3.1 and 4.1; Figure 3.1 and 4.1). This might indicate that thrombin at this dose is inactivated rapidly and therefore it can not exert its full pro-thrombotic action. However, as we did not measure the levels of thrombin-antithrombin complexes, we can not confirm this hypothesis.

Our study provides information regarding time-dependency of thrombin- induced changes in coagulation parameters (Figures 4.2 and 4.3). While thrombin decreased fibrinogen levels already one hour after start of infusion with a nadir at 3 hours (Figure 4.3A), maximal prolongation in thrombin time and aPTT was observed at 5 hours (Figures 4.3C and 4.3D). Interestingly, fibrinogen did not return to baseline during the study period, which is reflected by changes in maximum clot firmness (MCF) and alpha angle (Figure 4.6). Thrombin generation decreased after infusion of thrombin, likely due to consumption of coagulation factors such as FVIII (Figure 4.7B). Similar to fibrinogen, thrombin generation remained suppressed for 72 hours, but the assay measures formation of a chromogenic substrate and is not dependent on fibrinogen. Potentially, consumption of coagulation factors with a long half-life such as prothrombin (2.8 days) [184] may account for this observation.

While a thrombin – induced decrease in FVIII and FXIII (Figure 4.4) is likely explained by consumption of these factors by thrombin infusion, an increase in FV and FX

*Discussion*

activity is to our knowledge hitherto unreported. Whereas the increase in FV could be due to FV release from the alpha granules of activated platelets, we have no ready explanation for the 40% increase in FX. Yet the association between FV and FX is remarkable in view that FV is activated by FX 50-100 times more efficiently than by thrombin, and that FVa is a very effective cofactor for FXa [185].

In addition to a recognized role in the coagulation cascade and haemostasis, thrombin is known to have multiple pleiotropic functions. Although thrombin led to expression or secretion of MCP-1 [186], IL-10 [34], and TNF-alpha [37] in *in vitro* experiments, intravenous infusion of thrombin did not alter levels of those cytokines in our study, demonstrating that *in vitro* findings not always match the *in vivo* results. Thrombin is known to increase IL-6 levels *in vitro* [34,186,187] but *in vivo* data were lacking, although antithrombin decreased IL-6 formation in human endotoxemia [116]. Our study shows for the first time that thrombin increases only levels of IL-6 dose-dependently *in vivo* (Figure 3.1C), which might be mediated by the PAR-1 receptor [37]. Interestingly, the thrombin dose correlated with IL-6 levels better than with fibrinogen or platelet counts, which might be explained by counter-regulatory mechanisms inactivating many of the thrombin effects in coagulation and lack of such mechanisms if thrombin acts *via* the PAR-1 receptor. Increased levels of IL-6 are frequently observed in disseminated intravascular coagulation [179]. Interestingly, infusion of drotrecogin alfa (rhAPC) was associated with a relative decrease of IL-6 in septic patients although it had no effects on IL-6 in non-overt DIC during human endotoxemia [188].

In contrast, no change in the expression patterns of cytokines was observed in sheep when assessed by the proteomic analysis. This might be due to the fact that these proteins are present in too low levels to be seen on 2-DE gels. Cytokines, which in general act locally at the site of infection or inflammation, are not active at their normal plasma concentrations because they are diluted from microliter or milliliter volumes of tissue into 17 liters of interstitial fluid. Hence they are in a sense leakage markers as well, although their presence in plasma does not indicate cell breakage [189]. Secondly, changes in plasma proteins might not be detectable due to their rapid clearance or because products below the detectable size in the gel (about 10kD) are created. Thirdly, it is possible that small amounts of degradation products of some other proteins are largely overlapping in the 2-DE pattern with major spots, which makes them not recognizable as different proteins. Fourthly, the sensitivity of the proteomic analysis might not be sufficient to detect trace proteins which are affected in concentration. In 2-DE only proteins differing by up to two

## Discussion

orders of magnitude can be displayed on the same gel. For example, between the concentration of albumin and IL-6 are more than 10 orders of magnitude [189].

The effects of thrombin are in contrast to the human endotoxemia model, where an estimated thrombin generation of 0.4-0.8 IU/kg over 6 hours activates the coagulation system, transiently shortens the aPTT and prolongs the prothrombin time [190]. Endotoxin shortened clotting time (thromboelastometry) and closure times (PFA-100) in humans [114], which is in contrast to the effects of thrombin, which maximally prolonged both parameters (Figure 4.6). This indicates that while endotoxin displays strong pro-coagulant activity, anticoagulant properties of thrombin overweigh during its systemic infusion. The effect of thrombin on clotting time and clot formation time was reversible within 24 hours (Figure 4.6A). The patterns of aPTT resembled thromboelastometry, so that consumption of coagulation factors may have caused these changes. Additionally, prolongation of clotting time in thromboelastometry was associated with lung haemorrhage in all animals receiving the highest thrombin dose, indicating a good predictive value of this device for bleedings. Prolongation of the thrombin time can possibly be explained by the competition of fibrinogen degradation products and fibrinogen for the fibrinogen binding sites of thrombin [191] or delayed fibrin polymerization due to fibrin degradation products [192].

Intravenous endotoxin administration in rats caused thrombocytopenia and decrease in fibrinogen levels [193], which is similar to the effects of thrombin in our models of continuous thrombin infusion (Figure 3.1 and 4.2). A comparison of thrombin and endotoxin infusions in the same setting would be very helpful to characterise which effects are due to thrombin action and which are not.

Although the endotoxemia model can be a useful tool to study lipopolysacharide-induced tissue factor- triggered coagulation that can be used to characterise anticoagulants or anti-inflammatory drugs [190,194,195], it has several limitations: i) it fails to generate evidence of increased vascular permeability [196], ii) it does not reflect the pathophysiology of DIC during Gram-positive bacteraemia, and iii) the inflammation is prevailing.

An alternative model of inducing DIC is the systemic infusion of tissue factor. However, during infusion of tissue factor it is not possible to examine isolated thrombin effects, which was one major aim of the study. Accordingly, there are proteins, which are able to directly activate thrombin such as staphylocoagulase bypassing the usual tissue factor/factor VII/factor X pathway. However, to our knowledge, a model of staphylocoagulase- induced DIC has not been established yet. Although all these models

*Discussion*

have some degree of artificiality, we believe that our model could be an additional tool for investigating the effects of protracted thrombin exposure.

## 5.3. Limitations

Possible imprecision in study results could have arisen from limitations inherent to the laboratory assays used, which are standardised for human blood. Nevertheless, the NATEM test (Non-Activated Thrombelastometry) without any activator showed relevant differences between species. Different sensitivity of each species to the human thrombin is an inherent limitation of the study. A possible limitation for the comparison of the coagulation profile between humans and rats could be the blood sampling by heart puncture in rats, which could lead to positive test results for markers of coagulation activation due to tissue damage [197]. A limitation of the rat model might be high inter-individual variability in response to thrombin infusion observed in our study. Additionally, as ovine platelets might display differences in the expression of protease-activated receptors (PARs) as compared to human platelets, the impact of thrombin on thrombocytopenia in our model could be difficult to interpret. Moreover, proteomic studies have been carried out on plasma samples without prior depletion of highly abundant proteins. Although depletion is often recommended for serum/plasma samples, to achieve higher sensitivity due to removal of albumin, IgG, and sometimes also of several medium-abundant proteins, commercial reagents are only available for human specimens.

Our results show that only the haemorrhagic component of DIC could be mimicked in the animal models of continuous thrombin infusion at steady state conditions. DIC in humans often starts primarily as a thrombotic process, which becomes thrombo-hemorrhagic with time. The end-organ damage may occur during the early thrombotic phase, before levels of laboratory parameters of DIC become abnormal. The lack of evidence for end-organ damage in our study may suggest that systemic infusion of thrombin alone is not sufficient to produce DIC. Secondly, elevated markers of inflammation are seen in patients with diseases that are accompanied by DIC. The relatively sparse evidence for inflammation after thrombin infusion in this model might suggest that that protracted exposure to thrombin is not generating a process similar to disease-induced DIC.

# 6. CONCLUSIONS

There are relevant differences in the coagulation profile with or without thrombin stimulation between the five different species tested: humans, rats, sheep, pigs and rabbits. The cross-species comparison indicates that sheep could be a suitable species for translational coagulation studies. In addition, our findings confirm the usefulness of pigs as an experimental species for examining the fibrinolytic pathway and support the usefulness of rabbits as a species for studies on platelets. Although rats are widely used animal species in coagulation studies, our study showed that they are least comparable to humans. In sum, our findings indicate that precautions must be taken in the interpretation of the results and in extrapolation of animal studies to humans in the field of haemostasis because of marked species differences.

Protracted intravenous infusion of thrombin in sheep and rats over a period of five hours offers a new experimental model of consumption coagulopathy, where thrombin did not show pro-coagulant properties but lead to haemorrhage. Consumption of fibrinogen and platelets in our rat model correlated with bleeding events and mortality. In contrast to *in vitro* findings, the proinflammatory role of thrombin can only be confirmed for IL-6. These models can be further used to study isolated effects of thrombin *in vivo*.

# 7. REFERENCES

1. Gamgee A. On some old and new experiments on the fibrin-ferment. *The Journal of Physiology*. 1879:145-163.
2. Davie EW, Kulman JD. An overview of the structure and function of thrombin. *Semin Thromb Hemost*. 2006;32 Suppl 1:3-15.
3. Creasey AA, Reinhart K. Tissue factor pathway inhibitor activity in severe sepsis. *Crit Care Med*. 2001;29:S126-9.
4. Di Cera E. Thrombin as procoagulant and anticoagulant. *J Thromb Haemost*. 2007;5 Suppl 1:196-202.
5. Bode W. The structure of thrombin: a janus-headed proteinase. *Semin Thromb Hemost*. 2006;32 Suppl 1:16-31.
6. Qureshi SH, Yang L, Manithody C, Iakhiaev AV, Rezaie AR. Mutagenesis studies toward understanding allostery in thrombin. *Biochemistry*. 2009;48:8261-70.
7. Stubbs MT, Bode W. The clot thickens: clues provided by thrombin structure. *Trends Biochem Sci*. 1995;20:23-8.
8. Meeks SL, Abshire TC. Abnormalities of prothrombin: a review of the pathophysiology, diagnosis, and treatment. *Haemophilia*. 2008;14:1159-63.
9. Lancellotti S, De Cristofaro R. Congenital prothrombin deficiency. *Semin Thromb Hemost*. 2009;35:367-81.
10. Huang JN, Koerper MA. Factor V deficiency: a concise review. *Haemophilia*. 2008;14:1164-9.
11. Chen D, Dorling A. Critical roles for thrombin in acute and chronic inflammation. *J Thromb Haemost*. 2009;7 Suppl 1:122-6.
12. Suzuki H, Shima M, Nogami K, Sakurai Y, Nishiya K, Saenko EL, Tanaka I, Yoshioka A. Factor V C2 domain contains a major thrombin-binding site responsible for thrombin-catalyzed factor V activation. *J Thromb Haemost*. 2006;4:1354-60.
13. Fritsch P, Cvirn G, Cimenti C, Baier K, Gallistl S, Koestenberger M, Roschitz B, Leschnik B, Muntean W. Thrombin generation in factor VIII-depleted neonatal plasma: nearly normal because of physiologically low antithrombin and tissue factor pathway inhibitor. *J Thromb Haemost*. 2006;4:1071-7.
14. von dem Borne PA, Cox LM, Bouma BN. Factor XI enhances fibrin generation and inhibits fibrinolysis in a coagulation model initiated by surface-coated tissue factor. *Blood Coagul Fibrinolysis*. 2006;17:251-257.

*References*

15. Ponce RA, Visich JE, Heffernan JK, Lewis KB, Pederson S, Lebel E, Andrews-Jones L, Elliott G, Palmer TE, Rogge MC. Preclinical safety and pharmacokinetics of recombinant human factor XIII. *Toxicol Pathol*. 2005;33:495-506.

16. Lundblad RL, White GC, 2nd. The interaction of thrombin with blood platelets. *Platelets*. 2005;16:373-85.

17. Ozuyaman B, Godecke A, Kusters S, Kirchhoff E, Scharf RE, Schrader J. Endothelial nitric oxide synthase plays a minor role in inhibition of arterial thrombus formation. *Thromb Haemost*. 2005;93:1161-7.

18. Cleator JH, Zhu WQ, Vaughan DE, Hamm HE. Differential regulation of endothelial exocytosis of P-selectin and von Willebrand factor by protease-activated receptors and cAMP. *Blood*. 2006;107:2736-44.

19. George JN, Torres MM. Thrombin decreases von Willebrand factor binding to platelet glycoprotein Ib. *Blood*. 1988;71:1253-9.

20. Valnickova Z, Christensen T, Skottrup P, Thogersen IB, Hojrup P, Enghild JJ. Post-translational modifications of human thrombin-activatable fibrinolysis inhibitor (TAFI): evidence for a large shift in the isoelectric point and reduced solubility upon activation. *Biochemistry*. 2006;45:1525-35.

21. Brogren H, Karlsson L, Andersson M, Wang L, Erlinge D, Jern S. Platelets synthesize large amounts of active plasminogen activator inhibitor 1. *Blood*. 2004;104:3943-8.

22. Peterson EA, Sutherland MR, Nesheim ME, Pryzdial EL. Thrombin induces endothelial cell-surface exposure of the plasminogen receptor annexin 2. *J Cell Sci*. 2003;116:2399-408.

23. Rickles FR, Patierno S, Fernandez PM. Tissue factor, thrombin, and cancer. *Chest*. 2003;124:58S-68S.

24. Coughlin SR. Protease-activated receptors in hemostasis, thrombosis and vascular biology. *J Thromb Haemost*. 2005;3:1800-14.

25. Kahn ML, Nakanishi-Matsui M, Shapiro MJ, Ishihara H, Coughlin SR. Protease-activated receptors 1 and 4 mediate activation of human platelets by thrombin. *J Clin Invest*. 1999;103:879-87.

26. Kahn ML, Zheng YW, Huang W, Bigornia V, Zeng D, Moff S, Farese RV, Jr., Tam C, Coughlin SR. A dual thrombin receptor system for platelet activation. *Nature*. 1998;394:690-4.

27. Andrade-Gordon P, Derian CK, Maryanoff BE, Zhang HC, Addo MF, Cheung W, Damiano BP, D'Andrea MR, Darrow AL, de Garavilla L, Eckardt AJ, Giardino EC,

*References*

Haertlein BJ, McComsey DF. Administration of a potent antagonist of protease-activated receptor-1 (PAR-1) attenuates vascular restenosis following balloon angioplasty in rats. *J Pharmacol Exp Ther*. 2001;298:34-42.

28. Martorell L, Martinez-Gonzalez J, Rodriguez C, Gentile M, Calvayrac O, Badimon L. Thrombin and protease-activated receptors (PARs) in atherothrombosis. *Thromb Haemost*. 2008;99:305-15.

29. Camerer E, Cornelissen I, Kataoka H, Duong DN, Zheng YW, Coughlin SR. Roles of protease-activated receptors in a mouse model of endotoxemia. *Blood*. 2006;107:3912-21.

30. Kazerani HR, Plevin R, Kawagoe J, Kanke T, Furman BL. Lack of effect of proteinase-activated receptor-2 (PAR-2) deletion on the pathophysiological changes produced by lipopolysaccharide in the mouse: comparison with dexamethasone. *J Pharm Pharmacol*. 2004;56:1015-20.

31. Yaguchi A, Lobo FL, Vincent JL, Pradier O. Platelet function in sepsis. *J Thromb Haemost*. 2004;2:2096-102.

32. Pawlinski R, Mackman N. Tissue factor, coagulation proteases, and protease-activated receptors in endotoxemia and sepsis. *Crit Care Med*. 2004;32:S293-7.

33. Reiter R, Derhaschnig U, Spiel A, Keen P, Cardona F, Mayr F, Jilma B. Regulation of protease-activated receptor 1 (PAR1) on platelets and responsiveness to thrombin receptor activating peptide (TRAP) during systemic inflammation in humans. *Thromb Haemost*. 2003;90:898-903.

34. Esmon CT. The interactions between inflammation and coagulation. *Br J Haematol*. 2005;131:417-30.

35. Seybold J, Thomas D, Witzenrath M, Boral S, Hocke AC, Burger A, Hatzelmann A, Tenor H, Schudt C, Krull M, Schutte H, Hippenstiel S, Suttorp N. Tumor necrosis factor-alpha-dependent expression of phosphodiesterase 2: role in endothelial hyperpermeability. *Blood*. 2005;105:3569-76.

36. Zimmerman GA, Elstad MR, Lorant DE, McLntyre TM, Prescott SM, Topham MK, Weyrich AS, Whatley RE. Platelet-activating factor (PAF): signalling and adhesion in cell-cell interactions. *Adv Exp Med Biol*. 1996;416:297-304.

37. Fan Y, Zhang W, Mulholland M. Thrombin and PAR-1-AP increase proinflammatory cytokine expression in C6 cells. *J Surg Res*. 2005;129:196-201.

38. Cakmak H, Schatz F, Huang ST, Buchwalder L, Rahman M, Arici A, Lockwood CJ. Progestin suppresses thrombin- and interleukin-1beta-induced interleukin-11

*References*

production in term decidual cells: implications for preterm delivery. *J Clin Endocrinol Metab.* 2005;90:5279-86.

39. Naldini A, Bernini C, Pucci A, Carraro F. Thrombin-mediated IL-10 up-regulation involves protease-activated receptor (PAR)-1 expression in human mononuclear leukocytes. *J Leukoc Biol.* 2005;78:736-44.

40. Marklund M, Lerner UH, Persson M, Ransjo M. Bradykinin and thrombin stimulate release of arachidonic acid and formation of prostanoids in human periodontal ligament cells. *Eur J Orthod.* 1994;16:213-21.

41. Razin E, Marx G. Thrombin-induced degranulation of cultured bone marrow-derived mast cells. *J Immunol.* 1984;133:3282-5.

42. Miho N, Ishida T, Kuwaba N, Ishida M, Shimote-Abe K, Tabuchi K, Oshima T, Yoshizumi M, Chayama K. Role of the JNK pathway in thrombin-induced ICAM-1 expression in endothelial cells. *Cardiovasc Res.* 2005;68:289-98.

43. Szaba FM, Smiley ST. Roles for thrombin and fibrin(ogen) in cytokine/chemokine production and macrophage adhesion in vivo. *Blood.* 2002;99:1053-9.

44. Birukova AA, Birukov KG, Smurova K, Adyshev D, Kaibuchi K, Alieva I, Garcia JG, Verin AD. Novel role of microtubules in thrombin-induced endothelial barrier dysfunction. *Faseb J.* 2004;18:1879-90.

45. Caunt M, Hu L, Tang T, Brooks PC, Ibrahim S, Karpatkin S. Growth-regulated oncogene is pivotal in thrombin-induced angiogenesis. *Cancer Res.* 2006;66:4125-32.

46. Lampugnani MG, Colotta F, Polentarutti N, Pedenovi M, Mantovani A, Dejana E. Thrombin induces c-fos expression in cultured human endothelial cells by a $Ca^{2+}$-dependent mechanism. *Blood.* 1990;76:1173-80.

47. Marsden PA, Dorfman DM, Collins T, Brenner BM, Orkin SH, Ballermann BJ. Regulated expression of endothelin 1 in glomerular capillary endothelial cells. *Am J Physiol.* 1991;261:F117-25.

48. Sarno JL, Schatz F, Lockwood CJ, Huang ST, Taylor HS. Thrombin and interleukin-1beta regulate HOXA10 expression in human term decidual cells: implications for preterm labor. *J Clin Endocrinol Metab.* 2006;91:2366-72.

49. Bluteau G, Pilet P, Bourges X, Bilban M, Spaethe R, Daculsi G, Guicheux J. The modulation of gene expression in osteoblasts by thrombin coated on biphasic calcium phosphate ceramic. *Biomaterials.* 2006;27:2934-43.

*References*

50. Cao H, Dronadula N, Rao GN. Thrombin induces expression of FGF-2 via activation of PI3K-Akt-Fra-1 signaling axis leading to DNA synthesis and motility in vascular smooth muscle cells. *Am J Physiol Cell Physiol*. 2006;290:C172-82.
51. Beckett CS, Pennington K, McHowat J. Activation of MAPKs in thrombin-stimulated ventricular myocytes is dependent on Ca2+-independent PLA2. *Am J Physiol Cell Physiol*. 2006;290:C1350-4.
52. Tang H, Low B, Rutherford SA, Hao Q. Thrombin induces endocytosis of endoglin and type-II TGF-beta receptor and down-regulation of TGF-beta signaling in endothelial cells. *Blood*. 2005;105:1977-85.
53. Kanda Y, Watanabe Y. Thrombin-induced glucose transport via Src-p38 MAPK pathway in vascular smooth muscle cells. *Br J Pharmacol*. 2005;146:60-7.
54. Gorlach A, BelAiba RS, Hess J, Kietzmann T. Thrombin activates the p21-activated kinase in pulmonary artery smooth muscle cells. Role in tissue factor expression. *Thromb Haemost*. 2005;93:1168-75.
55. Shankar H, Garcia A, Prabhakar J, Kim S, Kunapuli SP. P2Y12 receptor-mediated potentiation of thrombin-induced thromboxane A2 generation in platelets occurs through regulation of Erk1/2 activation. *J Thromb Haemost*. 2006;4:638-47.
56. Jennings LK. Mechanisms of platelet activation: need for new strategies to protect against platelet-mediated atherothrombosis. *Thromb Haemost*. 2009;102:248-57.
57. Ruggeri ZM, Zarpellon A, Roberts JR, McClintock RA, Jing H, Mendolicchio GL. Unravelling the mechanism and significance of thrombin binding to platelet glycoprotein Ib. *Thromb Haemost*. 2010;104:894-902.
58. Tsopanoglou NE, Maragoudakis ME. Role of thrombin in angiogenesis and tumor progression. *Semin Thromb Hemost*. 2004;30:63-9.
59. Ten Cate H. Trombocytopenia: one of the markers of disseminated intravascular coagulation. *Pathophysiol Haemost Thromb*. 2003;33:413-6.
60. Toh CH, Dennis M. Disseminated intravascular coagulation: old disease, new hope. *Bmj*. 2003;327:974-7.
61. Dhainaut JF, Yan SB, Joyce DE, Pettila V, Basson B, Brandt JT, Sundin DP, Levi M. Treatment effects of drotrecogin alfa (activated) in patients with severe sepsis with or without overt disseminated intravascular coagulation. *J Thromb Haemost*. 2004;2:1924-33.
62. Colvin BT. Physiology of haemostasis. *Vox Sang*. 2004;87 Suppl1:43-6.
63. Owens AP, 3rd, Mackman N. Tissue factor and thrombosis: The clot starts here. *Thromb Haemost*. 2010;104:432-9.

*References*

64. Levi M, Ten Cate H. Disseminated intravascular coagulation. *N Engl J Med.* 1999;341:586-92.

65. Momi S, Nasimi M, Colucci M, Nenci GG, Gresele P. Low molecular weight heparins prevent thrombin-induced thrombo-embolism in mice despite low anti-thrombin activity. Evidence that the inhibition of feed-back activation of thrombin generation confers safety advantages over direct thrombin inhibition. *Haematologica.* 2001;86:297-302.

66. Ballabeni V, Calcina F, Tognolini M, Bruno O, Manotti C, Barocelli E. Effects of subacute treatment with benzopyranopyrimidines in hemostasis and experimental thrombosis in mice. *Life Sci.* 2004;74:1851-9.

67. Gresele P, Momi S, Berrettini M, Nenci GG, Schwarz HP, Semeraro N, Colucci M. Activated human protein C prevents thrombin-induced thromboembolism in mice. Evidence that activated protein c reduces intravascular fibrin accumulation through the inhibition of additional thrombin generation. *J Clin Invest.* 1998;101:667-76.

68. Margaretten W, Zunker HO, McKay DG. Production of the Generalized Shwartzman Reaction in Pregnant Rats by Intravenous Infusion of Thrombin. *Lab Invest.* 1964;13:552-9.

69. Kaplan JE, Snedeker PW, Baum SH, Moon DG, Minnear FL. Influence of plasma fibronectin on the response to infusion of thrombin and adenosine diphosphate. *Thromb Haemost.* 1983;49:217-23.

70. Witte S, Schricker KT. [The behavior of the blood vessels in experimental hemostasis.]. *Z Gesamte Exp Med.* 1960;133:361-74.

71. Gorog P, Kovacs IB. Increase in bronchial resistance during infusion of thrombin into the venous circulation of guinea pigs. Improved model for experimental pulmonary microembolism. *Angiologica.* 1973;10:164-72.

72. Colucci M, Triggiani R, Cavallo LG, Semeraro N. Thrombin infusion in endotoxin-treated rabbits reduces the plasma levels of plasminogen activator inhibitor: evidence for a protein-C-mediated mechanism. *Blood.* 1989;74:1976-82.

73. Davis RB, Palmer MJ. Thrombocytopenia and release of platelet amines induced by thrombin and bacterial lipopolysaccharide. Observations after infusion of low molecular weight dextran. *Br J Exp Pathol.* 1965;46:554-63.

74. Burchardi H, Stokke T, Hensel I, Kostering H, Rahlf G, Schlag G, Heine H, Horl WH. Adult respiratory distress syndrome (ARDS): experimental models with elastase and thrombin infusion in pigs. *Adv Exp Med Biol.* 1984;167:319-33.

## References

75. Bennett JM, Yu D, Suyemoto J, Pechet L. The effects of infusing thrombin and its acetylated derivative. II. Observations on intravascular hemolysis with pathologic correlations. *Thromb Diath Haemorrh*. 1968;20:469-76.
76. Nordstrom S, Zetterqvist E. Effects of thrombin infusions upon 131-I-labelled fibrinogen in dogs. *Acta Physiol Scand*. 1968;72:85-99.
77. Whitaker AN, McKay DG. Induction of hypotension in rhesus monkeys and rabbits by intravenous thrombin infusion. *Lab Invest*. 1969;20:79-86.
78. Lentz SR, Fernandez JA, Griffin JH, Piegors DJ, Erger RA, Malinow MR, Heistad DD. Impaired anticoagulant response to infusion of thrombin in atherosclerotic monkeys associated with acquired defects in the protein C system. *Arterioscler Thromb Vasc Biol*. 1999;19:1744-50.
79. Arfors KE, Busch C, Jakobson S, Lindquist O, Malmberg P, Rammer L, Saldeen T. Pulmonary insufficiency following intravenous infusion of thrombin and AMCA (tranexamic acid) in the dog. *Acta Chir Scand*. 1972;138:445-52.
80. Girolami A, Cliffton EE, Agostino D. Hemorrhagic syndrome in dogs induced by intravenous thrombin. *Thromb Diath Haemorrh*. 1966;16:243-56.
81. Lee L. Reticuloendothelial clearance of circulating fibrin in the pathogenesis of the generalized Shwartzman reaction. *J Exp Med*. 1962;115:1065-82.
82. Quick AJ, Hussey CV, Harris J, Peters K. Occult intravascular clotting by means of intravenous injection of thrombin. *Am J Physiol*. 1959;197:791-4.
83. Delin A, Olsson P, Teger-Nilsson AC. Vasodilatation in the canine leg caused by intraarterial infusion of thrombin and tissue thromboplastin. *Cardiovasc Res*. 1967;1:371-8.
84. Siller-Matula JM, Bayer G, Bergmeister H, Quehenberger P, Petzelbauer P, Friedl P, Mesteri I, Jilma B. An experimental model to study isolated effects of thrombin in vivo. *Thromb Res*. 2010;126:454-61.
85. Monkhouse FC, Milojevic S. Changes in fibrinogen level after infusion of thrombin and thromboplastin. *Am J Physiol*. 1960;199:1165-8.
86. Soulier JP, Gozin D, Lerable J. In vivo attempt to consume antithrombin III by i.v. injection of a thrombin-heparin mixture. *Thromb Res*. 1984;34:255-62.
87. Unruh M, Grunow A, Gottstein C. Systemic coagulation parameters in mice after treatment with vascular targeting agents. *Thromb J*. 2005;3:21.
88. Ro JS, Flatmark A. Studies on thrombin infusion in dogs. *Scand J Haematol*. 1972;9:293-304.

## References

89. Kowalski E, Budzynski AZ, Kopec M, Latallo ZS, Lipinski B, Wegrzynowicz Z. Circulating Fibrinogen Degradation Products (Fdp) in Dog Blood after Intravenous Thrombin Infusion. *Thromb Diath Haemorrh*. 1965;13:12-24.
90. Jastrzebski J, Arnot RN, Hilgard P, Sykes MK. Thrombin-induced disseminated intravascular coagulation in the dog. I: Demonstration of microthrombi in lung. *Br J Anaesth*. 1975;47:654-7.
91. Jastrzebski J, Hilgard P, Chakrabarti MK, Henry K, Sykes MK. Thrombin-induced disseminated intravascular coagulation in the dog. II. Cardiorespiratory changes during spontaneous and controlled ventilation. *Br J Anaesth*. 1975;47:658-65.
92. Kumada T, Dittman WA, Majerus PW. A role for thrombomodulin in the pathogenesis of thrombin-induced thromboembolism in mice. *Blood*. 1988;71:728-33.
93. Radegran K, Cronestrand R, Olsson P. The effect of regional thrombin infusion on the renal vascular resistance. *Eur Surg Res*. 1970;2:460-70.
94. Chen B, Cheng Q, Yang K, Lyden PD. Thrombin Mediates Severe Neurovascular Injury During Ischemia. *Stroke*. 2010.
95. Nagase H, Kitazato KT, Sasaki E, Hattori M, Kitazato K, Saito H. Antithrombin III-independent effect of depolymerized holothurian glycosaminoglycan (DHG) on acute thromboembolism in mice. *Thromb Haemost*. 1997;77:399-402.
96. Collins RD, Robbins BH, Mayes CE. Studies on the pathogenesis of the generalized Shwartzman reaction. Production of glomerular thrombosis and renal cortical necrosis by intraaortic thrombin infusion in normal and leucopenic rabbits. *Johns Hopkins Med J*. 1968;122:375-9.
97. Stafford BT, Rapaport SI, Shen SM. The effects of infusion of thrombin or endotoxin in rabbits treated with cortisone. *Thromb Diath Haemorrh*. 1975;34:159-68.
98. Geier B, Muth-Werthmann D, Barbera L, Bolle I, Militzer K, Philippou S, Mumme A. Laparoscopic ligation of the infrarenal vena cava in combination with transfemoral thrombin infusion: a new animal model of chronic deep venous thrombosis. *Eur J Vasc Endovasc Surg*. 2005;29:542-8.
99. Hoie J, Schenk WG, Jr. Experimental intravascular coagulation: impairment of renal blood flow following thrombin infusion in the dog. *J Trauma*. 1972;12:302-8.
100. Busch C, Lindquist O, Saldeen T. Effect of reptilase on respiratory insufficiency induced by intravenous infusion of thrombin and AMCA (tranexamic acid) in the dog. *Bibl Anat*. 1973;12:254-9.

*References*

101. Lindquist O, Malmberg P. Heart lymph flow and aspartate aminotransferase activity after infusion of thrombin and tranexamic acid in the dog. *Scand J Clin Lab Invest.* 1972;30:145-51.
102. Lundblad RL, Bradshaw RA, Gabriel D, Ortel TL, Lawson J, Mann KG. A review of the therapeutic uses of thrombin. *Thromb Haemost.* 2004;91:851-60.
103. He Z, Hoppensteadt D, Cunanan J, Fareed J. Cross-reactivity of rabbit anti-bovine thrombin IgGs with human alpha-thrombin and a recombinant version of human thrombin (Recothrom). *Clin Appl Thromb Hemost.* 2010;16:273-80.
104. Di Nisio M, Middeldorp S, Buller HR. Direct thrombin inhibitors. *N Engl J Med.* 2005;353:1028-40.
105. Becker DL, Fredenburgh JC, Stafford AR, Weitz JI. Exosites 1 and 2 are essential for protection of fibrin-bound thrombin from heparin-catalyzed inhibition by antithrombin and heparin cofactor II. *J Biol Chem.* 1999;274:6226-33.
106. Kalus JS, Caron MF. Novel uses for current and future direct thrombin inhibitors: focus on ximelagatran and bivalirudin. *Expert Opin Investig Drugs.* 2004;13:465-77.
107. Schaden E, Kozek-Langenecker SA. Direct thrombin inhibitors: pharmacology and application in intensive care medicine. *Intensive Care Med*;36:1127-37.
108. Laterre PF, Wittebole X, Collienne C. Pharmacological inhibition of tissue factor. *Semin Thromb Hemost.* 2006;32:71-6.
109. Perel P, Roberts I, Sena E, Wheble P, Briscoe C, Sandercock P, Macleod M, Mignini LE, Jayaram P, Khan KS. Comparison of treatment effects between animal experiments and clinical trials: systematic review. *Bmj.* 2007;334:197.
110. Siller-Matula JM, Jilma B. Strain differences in toxic effects of long-lasting isoflurane anaesthesia between Wistar rats and Sprague Dawley rats. *Food Chem Toxicol.* 2008;46:3550-2.
111. Saito K, Sakai N, Kim HS, Ishizuka M, Kazusaka A, Fujita S. Strain differences in diazepam metabolism at its three metabolic sites in sprague-dawley, brown norway, dark agouti, and wistar strain rats. *Drug Metab Dispos.* 2004;32:959-65.
112. Walberer M, Stolz E, Muller C, Friedrich C, Rottger C, Blaes F, Kaps M, Fisher M, Bachmann G, Gerriets T. Experimental stroke: ischaemic lesion volume and oedema formation differ among rat strains (a comparison between Wistar and Sprague-Dawley rats using MRI). *Lab Anim.* 2006;40:1-8.
113. Luddington RJ. Thrombelastography/thromboelastometry. *Clin Lab Haematol.* 2005;27:81-90.

*References*

114. Spiel AO, Mayr FB, Firbas C, Quehenberger P, Jilma B. Validation of rotation thrombelastography in a model of systemic activation of fibrinolysis and coagulation in humans. *J Thromb Haemost.* 2006;4:411-6.
115. Lang T, Bauters A, Braun SL, Potzsch B, von Pape KW, Kolde HJ, Lakner M. Multi-centre investigation on reference ranges for ROTEM thromboelastometry. *Blood Coagul Fibrinolysis.* 2005;16:301-10.
116. Leitner JM, Firbas C, Mayr FB, Reiter RA, Steinlechner B, Jilma B. Recombinant human antithrombin inhibits thrombin formation and interleukin 6 release in human endotoxemia. *Clin Pharmacol Ther.* 2006;79:23-34.
117. Anderson L, Quasim I, Soutar R, Steven M, Macfie A, Korte W. An audit of red cell and blood product use after the institution of thromboelastometry in a cardiac intensive care unit. *Transfus Med.* 2006;16:31-9.
118. Craft RM, Chavez JJ, Bresee SJ, Wortham DC, Cohen E, Carroll RC. A novel modification of the Thrombelastograph assay, isolating platelet function, correlates with optical platelet aggregation. *J Lab Clin Med.* 2004;143:301-9.
119. Siller-Matula JM, Plasenzotti R, Spiel A, Quehenberger P, Jilma B. Interspecies differences in coagulation profile. *Thromb Haemost.* 2008;100:397-404.
120. Jilma B. Platelet function analyzer (PFA-100): a tool to quantify congenital or acquired platelet dysfunction. *J Lab Clin Med.* 2001;138:152-63.
121. Siller-Matula JM, Haberl K, Prillinger K, Panzer S, Lang I, Jilma B. The effect of antiplatelet drugs clopidogrel and aspirin is less immediately after stent implantation. *Thromb Res.* 2009;123:874-80.
122. Siller-Matula JM, Gouya G, Wolzt M, Jilma B. Cross validation of the Multiple Electrode Aggregometry. A prospective trial in healthy volunteers. *Thromb Haemost.* 2009;102:397-403.
123. Siller-Matula JM, Spiel AO, Lang IM, Kreiner G, Christ G, Jilma B. Effects of pantoprazole and esomeprazole on platelet inhibition by clopidogrel. *Am Heart J.* 2009;157:148 e1-5.
124. Jilma B, Paulinska P, Jilma-Stohlawetz P, Gilbert JC, Hutabarat R, Knobl P. A randomised pilot trial of the anti-von Willebrand factor aptamer ARC1779 in patients with type 2b von Willebrand disease. *Thromb Haemost.* 2010;104:563-70.
125. Marouga R, David S, Hawkins E. The development of the DIGE system: 2D fluorescence difference gel analysis technology. *Anal Bioanal Chem.* 2005;382:669-78.

*References*

126. Miller I, Radwan M, Strobl B, Muller M, Gemeiner M. Contribution of cell culture additives to the two-dimensional protein patterns of mouse macrophages. *Electrophoresis*. 2006;27:1626-9.

127. Gutierrez AM, Miller I, Hummel K, Nobauer K, Martinez-Subiela S, Razzazi-Fazeli E, Gemeiner M, Ceron JJ. Proteomic analysis of porcine saliva. *Vet J*. 2010:doi:10.1016/j.tvjl.2009.12.020.

128. Lasserre JP, Fack F, Revets D, Planchon S, Renaut J, Hoffmann L, Gutleb AC, Muller CP, Bohn T. Effects of the endocrine disruptors atrazine and PCB 153 on the protein expression of MCF-7 human cells. *J Proteome Res*. 2009;8:5485-96.

129. Clauss A. [Rapid physiological coagulation method in determination of fibrinogen.]. *Acta Haematol*. 1957;17:237-46.

130. Langdell RD, Wagner RH, Brinkhous KM. Effect of antihemophilic factor on one-stage clotting tests; a presumptive test for hemophilia and a simple one-stage antihemophilic factor assy procedure. *J Lab Clin Med*. 1953;41:637-47.

131. Speiser W, Kapiotis S, Kopp CW, Simonitsch I, Jilma B, Jansen B, Exner M, Chott A. Effect of intradermal tumor necrosis factor-alpha-induced inflammation on coagulation factors in dermal vessel endothelium. An in vivo study of human skin biopsies. *Thromb Haemost*. 2001;85:362-7.

132. Konstantinides S, Schafer K, Neels JG, Dellas C, Loskutoff DJ. Inhibition of endogenous leptin protects mice from arterial and venous thrombosis. *Arterioscler Thromb Vasc Biol*. 2004;24:2196-201.

133. Miller I, Gianazza E, Gemeiner M. Any use in proteomics for low-tech approaches? Detecting fibrinogen chains of different animal species in two-dimensional electrophoresis patterns. *J Chromatogr B Analyt Technol Biomed Life Sci*. 2010;878:2314-8.

134. Flight SM, Masci PP, Lavin MF, Gaffney PJ. Resistance of porcine blood clots to lysis relates to poor activation of porcine plasminogen by tissue plasminogen activator. *Blood Coagul Fibrinolysis*. 2006;17:417-20.

135. Derian CK, Santulli RJ, Tomko KA, Haertlein BJ, Andrade-Gordon P. Species differences in platelet responses to thrombin and SFLLRN. receptor-mediated calcium mobilization and aggregation, and regulation by protein kinases. *Thromb Res*. 1995;78:505-19.

136. Sidhu P, Sutherland SB, Ganguly P. Interaction of thrombin with mammalian platelets. *Am J Physiol*. 1979;237:H353-8.

*References*

137. Nylander S, Mattsson C, Lindahl TL. Characterisation of species differences in the platelet ADP and thrombin response. *Thromb Res.* 2006;117:543-9.
138. Mosnier LO, Bouma BN. Regulation of fibrinolysis by thrombin activatable fibrinolysis inhibitor, an unstable carboxypeptidase B that unites the pathways of coagulation and fibrinolysis. *Arterioscler Thromb Vasc Biol.* 2006;26:2445-53.
139. Wu KK. Soluble thrombomodulin and coronary heart disease. *Curr Opin Lipidol.* 2003;14:373-5.
140. Bajzar L, Nesheim M, Morser J, Tracy PB. Both cellular and soluble forms of thrombomodulin inhibit fibrinolysis by potentiating the activation of thrombin-activable fibrinolysis inhibitor. *J Biol Chem.* 1998;273:2792-8.
141. Wielders S, Mukherjee M, Michiels J, Rijkers DT, Cambus JP, Knebel RW, Kakkar V, Hemker HC, Beguin S. The routine determination of the endogenous thrombin potential, first results in different forms of hyper- and hypocoagulability. *Thromb Haemost.* 1997;77:629-36.
142. Andrew M, Ofosu F, Fernandez F, Jefferies A, Hirsh J, Mitchell L, Buchanan MR. A low molecular weight heparin alters the fetal coagulation system in the pregnant sheep. *Thromb Haemost.* 1986;55:342-6.
143. Connell JM, Khalapyan T, Al-Mondhiry HA, Wilson RP, Rosenberg G, Weiss WJ. Anticoagulation of juvenile sheep and goats with heparin, warfarin, and clopidogrel. *Asaio J.* 2007;53:229-37.
144. Mottaghy K, Oedekoven B, Poppel K, Bruchmuller K, Kovacs B, Spahn A, Geisen C. Heparin free long-term extracorporeal circulation using bioactive surfaces. *ASAIO Trans.* 1989;35:635-7.
145. Hoehle P. Zur Übertragbarkeit tierexperimenteller endovaskulärer Studien: Unterschiede der Gerinnungs- und Fibrinolyse-Systeme bei häufig verwendeten Tierspezies im Vergleich zum Menschen. *Thesis.* 2000;RWTH Aachen University, Germany.
146. Berny PJ, de Oliveira LA, Videmann B, Rossi S. Assessment of ruminal degradation, oral bioavailability, and toxic effects of anticoagulant rodenticides in sheep. *Am J Vet Res.* 2006;67:363-71.
147. Oedekoven B, Bey R, Mottaghy K, Schmid-Schonbein H. Gabexate mesilate (Foy) as an anticoagulant in extracorporeal circulation in dogs and sheep. *Thromb Haemost.* 1984;52:329-32.

*References*

148. Shen LL, Barlow GH, Holleman WH. Differential activities of heparins in human plasma and in sheep plasma. Effects of heparin molecular sizes and sources. *Thromb Res.* 1978;13:671-9.

149. van Hylckama Vlieg A, Christiansen SC, Luddington R, Cannegieter SC, Rosendaal FR, Baglin TP. Elevated endogenous thrombin potential is associated with an increased risk of a first deep venous thrombosis but not with the risk of recurrence. *Br J Haematol.* 2007;138:769-74.

150. Karges HE, Funk KA, Ronneberger H. Activity of coagulation and fibrinolysis parameters in animals. *Arzneimittelforschung.* 1994;44:793-7.

151. Tillman P, Carson SN, Talken L. Platelet function and coagulation parameters in sheep during experimental vascular surgery. *Lab Anim Sci.* 1981;31:263-7.

152. Massicotte P, Mitchell L, Andrew M. A comparative study of coagulation systems in newborn animals. *Pediatr Res.* 1986;20:961-5.

153. Addonizio VP, Jr., Edmunds LH, Jr., Colman RW. The function of monkey (M. mulatta) platelets compared to platelets of pig, sheep, and man. *J Lab Clin Med.* 1978;91:989-97.

154. Burke SE, Lefer AM, Nicolaou KC, Smith GM, Smith JB. Responsiveness of platelets and coronary arteries from different species to synthetic thromboxane and prostaglandin endoperoxide analogues. *Br J Pharmacol.* 1983;78:287-92.

155. Read MS, Potter JY, Brinkhous KM. Venom coagglutinin for detection of von Willebrand factor activity in animal plasmas. *J Lab Clin Med.* 1983;101:74-82.

156. Prince MR, Salzman EW, Schoen FJ, Palestrant AM, Simon M. Local intravascular effects of the nitinol wire blood clot filter. *Invest Radiol.* 1988;23:294-300.

157. Grabowski EF, Didisheim P, Lewis JC, Franta JT, Stropp JQ. Platelet adhesion to foreign surfaces under controlled conditions of whole blood flow: human vs rabbit, dog, calf, sheep, pig, macaque, and baboon. *Trans Am Soc Artif Intern Organs.* 1977;23:141-51.

158. Hara T, Yokoyama A, Morishima Y, Kunitada S. Species differences in anticoagulant and anti-Xa activity of DX-9065a, a highly selective factor Xa inhibitor. *Thromb Res.* 1995;80:99-104.

159. Niitsu Y, Jakubowski JA, Sugidachi A, Asai F. Pharmacology of CS-747 (prasugrel, LY640315), a novel, potent antiplatelet agent with in vivo P2Y12 receptor antagonist activity. *Semin Thromb Hemost.* 2005;31:184-94.

*References*

160. Bijnens AP, Knockaert I, Cousin E, Kruithof EK, Declerck PJ. Expression and characterization of recombinant porcine plasminogen activator inhibitor-1. *Thromb Haemost*. 1997;77:350-6.
161. Marbet GA, Eichlisberger R, Duckert F, Ritz R, da Silva MA, Biland L, Widmer LK, Schmitt HE. Side effects of thrombolytic treatment with porcine plasmin and low dose streptokinase. *Thromb Haemost*. 1982;48:196-200.
162. Cliffton EE, Cannamela DA. Proteolytic and fibrinolytic activity of serum; activation by streptokinase and staphylokinase indicating dissimilarity of enzymes. *Blood*. 1953;8:554-62.
163. Thiex R, Kuker W, Muller HD, Rohde I, Schroder JM, Gilsbach JM, Rohde V. The long-term effect of recombinant tissue-plasminogen-activator (rt-PA) on edema formation in a large-animal model of intracerebral hemorrhage. *Neurol Res*. 2003;25:254-62.
164. Hardaway RM, Williams CH, Marvasti M, Farias M, Tseng A, Pinon I, Yanez D, Martinez M, Navar J. Prevention of adult respiratory distress syndrome with plasminogen activator in pigs. *Crit Care Med*. 1990;18:1413-8.
165. Vasquez Y, Williams CH, Hardaway RM. Effect of urokinase on disseminated intravascular coagulation. *J Appl Physiol*. 1998;85:1421-8.
166. Jern C, Seeman-Lodding H, Biber B, Winso O, Jern S. An experimental multiple-organ model for the study of regional net release/uptake rates of tissue-type plasminogen activator in the intact pig. *Thromb Haemost*. 1997;78:1150-6.
167. Nyberg A, Jakob SM, Seeman-Lodding H, Porta F, Bracht H, Bischofberger H, Jern C, Takala J, Aneman A. Time- and dose-related regional fluxes of tissue-type plasminogen activator in anesthetized endotoxemic pigs. *Acta Anaesthesiol Scand*. 2008;52:57-64.
168. McBane RD, 2nd, Ford MA, Karnicki K, Stewart M, Owen WG. Fibrinogen, fibrin and crosslinking in aging arterial thrombi. *Thromb Haemost*. 2000;84:83-7.
169. Gurbel PA, Bliden KP, Guyer K, Cho PW, Zaman KA, Kreutz RP, Bassi AK, Tantry US. Platelet reactivity in patients and recurrent events post-stenting: results of the PREPARE POST-STENTING Study. *J Am Coll Cardiol*. 2005;46:1820-6.
170. Hoefer IE, Grundmann S, Schirmer S, van Royen N, Meder B, Bode C, Piek JJ, Buschmann IR. Aspirin, but not clopidogrel, reduces collateral conductance in a rabbit model of femoral artery occlusion. *J Am Coll Cardiol*. 2005;46:994-1001.

## References

171. Golino P, Ambrosio G, Pascucci I, Ragni M, Russolillo E, Chiariello M. Experimental carotid stenosis and endothelial injury in the rabbit: an in vivo model to study intravascular platelet aggregation. *Thromb Haemost.* 1992;67:302-5.
172. van Gestel MA, Heemskerk JW, Slaaf DW, Heijnen VV, Reneman RS, oude Egbrink MG. In vivo blockade of platelet ADP receptor P2Y12 reduces embolus and thrombus formation but not thrombus stability. *Arterioscler Thromb Vasc Biol.* 2003;23:518-23.
173. van Giezen JJ, Humphries RG. Preclinical and clinical studies with selective reversible direct P2Y12 antagonists. *Semin Thromb Hemost.* 2005;31:195-204.
174. Greenbaum AB, Ohman EM, Gibson CM, Borzak S, Stebbins AL, Lu M, Le May MR, Stankowski JE, Emanuelsson H, Weaver WD. Preliminary experience with intravenous P2Y12 platelet receptor inhibition as an adjunct to reduced-dose alteplase during acute myocardial infarction: results of the Safety, Tolerability and Effect on Patency in Acute Myocardial Infarction (STEP-AMI) angiographic trial. *Am Heart J.* 2007;154:702-9.
175. Siller-Matula J, Schror K, Wojta J, Huber K. Thienopyridines in cardiovascular disease: focus on clopidogrel resistance. *Thromb Haemost.* 2007;97:385-93.
176. Ngo TH, Declerck PJ. Immunological quantitation of rabbit plasminogen activator inhibitor-1 in biological samples: evidence that rabbit platelets do not contain PAI-1. *Thromb Haemost.* 1999;82:1510-5.
177. Margaretten W, Csavossy I, McKay DG. An electron microscopic study of thrombin-induced disseminated intravascular coagulation. *Blood.* 1967;29:169-81.
178. Dempfle CE. Coagulopathy of sepsis. *Thromb Haemost.* 2004;91:213-24.
179. Levi M. Disseminated intravascular coagulation. *Crit Care Med.* 2007;35:2191-5.
180. Hanson SR, Griffin JH, Harker LA, Kelly AB, Esmon CT, Gruber A. Antithrombotic effects of thrombin-induced activation of endogenous protein C in primates. *J Clin Invest.* 1993;92:2003-12.
181. van Hinsbergh VW, Bertina RM, van Wijngaarden A, van Tilburg NH, Emeis JJ, Haverkate F. Activated protein C decreases plasminogen activator-inhibitor activity in endothelial cell-conditioned medium. *Blood.* 1985;65:444-51.
182. Vogel SM, Gao X, Mehta D, Ye RD, John TA, Andrade-Gordon P, Tiruppathi C, Malik AB. Abrogation of thrombin-induced increase in pulmonary microvascular permeability in PAR-1 knockout mice. *Physiol Genomics.* 2000;4:137-145.
183. Rice TW, Wheeler AP. Coagulopathy in critically ill patients: part 1: platelet disorders. *Chest.* 2009;136:1622-30.

*References*

184. Shapiro SS, Martinez J. Human prothrombin metabolism in normal man and in hypocoagulable subjects. *J Clin Invest*. 1969;48:1292-8.
185. Duckers C, Simioni P, Rosing J, Castoldi E. Advances in understanding the bleeding diathesis in factor V deficiency. *Br J Haematol*. 2009;146:17-26.
186. Marin V, Montero-Julian FA, Gres S, Boulay V, Bongrand P, Farnarier C, Kaplanski G. The IL-6-soluble IL-6Ralpha autocrine loop of endothelial activation as an intermediate between acute and chronic inflammation: an experimental model involving thrombin. *J Immunol*. 2001;167:3435-42.
187. Strande JL, Phillips SA. Thrombin increases inflammatory cytokine and angiogenic growth factor secretion in human adipose cells in vitro. *J Inflamm (Lond)*. 2009;6:4.
188. Derhaschnig U, Reiter R, Knobl P, Baumgartner M, Keen P, Jilma B. Recombinant human activated protein C (rhAPC; drotrecogin alfa [activated]) has minimal effect on markers of coagulation, fibrinolysis, and inflammation in acute human endotoxemia. *Blood*. 2003;102:2093-8.
189. Anderson NL, Anderson NG. The human plasma proteome: history, character, and diagnostic prospects. *Mol Cell Proteomics*. 2002;1:845-67.
190. Mayr FB, Jilma B. Coagulation interventions in experimental human endotoxemia. *Transl Res*. 2006;148:263-71.
191. Mischke R, Wolling H. Influence of fibrinogen degradation products on thrombin time, activated partial thromboplastin time and prothrombin time of canine plasma. *Haemostasis*. 2000;30:123-30.
192. Barth A, Furlan M, Lammle B. [Unexpectedly prolonged thrombin time]. *Schweiz Med Wochenschr*. 1993;123:523-9.
193. Iba T, Nakarai E, Takayama T, Nakajima K, Sasaoka T, Ohno Y. Combination effect of antithrombin and recombinant human soluble thrombomodulin in a lipopolysaccharide induced rat sepsis model. *Crit Care*. 2009;13:R203.
194. Derhaschnig U, Bergmair D, Marsik C, Schlifke I, Wijdenes J, Jilma B. Effect of interleukin-6 blockade on tissue factor-induced coagulation in human endotoxemia. *Crit Care Med*. 2004;32:1136-40.
195. Hollenstein U, Homoncik M, Knobl P, Pernerstorfer T, Graggaber J, Eichler HG, Handler S, Jilma B. Acenocoumarol decreases tissue factor-dependent coagulation during systemic inflammation in humans. *Clin Pharmacol Ther*. 2002;71:368-74.
196. Anel R, Kumar A. Human endotoxemia and human sepsis: limits to the model. *Crit Care*. 2005;9:151-2.

*References*

197. Unruh M, Grunow A, Gottstein C. Systemic coagulation parameters in mice after treatment with vascular targeting agents. *Thromb J.* 2005;3:21.

# LIST OF ABBREVIATIONS

| | |
|---|---|
| (-/-) | knock out |
| (+/+) | wild type |
| 2-DE | two-dimensional electrophoresis |
| Ang-2 | angiopoietin-2 |
| ALP | alkaline phosphatase |
| ALT | alanine aminotransferase |
| ANOVA | analysis of Variance |
| APC | activated protein C |
| APTT | activated partial thromboplastin time |
| ATIII | antithrombin III |
| AUC | area under the curve |
| BUN | blood urea nitrogen |
| CADP | collagen/adenosine diphosphate |
| CRP | C reactive protein |
| CT | clotting time |
| CFT | clot formation time |
| CVD | cardiovascular diseases |
| CXCR2 | chemokine receptor CXC |
| DIC | disseminated intravascular coagulation |
| DIGE | difference in gel electrophoresis |
| EC50 | half maximal effective concentration |
| ECG | electrocardiogram |
| EDTA | ethylenediaminetetra acetic acid |
| Erk1/2 | mitogen-activated protein kinase |
| ET | endothelin |
| ETP | endogenous thrombin potential |
| $F_{1+2}$ | prothrombin fragments |
| FDP | fibrin degradation products |
| FGF-2 | fibroblast growth factor-2 |
| GP | glycoprotein |
| GRO-alpha | growth-regulated oncogene-alpha |
| H&E | hematoxylin-and-eosin |
| HOXA10 | homeobox gene transcription factor |
| ICAM-1 | intercellular adhesion molecule 1 |

## List of abbreviations

| | |
|---|---|
| IL | interleukin |
| KDR | vascular endothelial growth factor receptor 2 |
| LD50 | lethal dose, at which 50% of subjects will die |
| LDH | lactate dehydrogenase |
| LMWH | low molecular weight heparin |
| LOAEL | lowest observed adverse effect level |
| LPS | lipopolysaccharide |
| MALDI-TOF/TOF | matrix assisted laser desorption ionization tandem time of flight |
| MAPK | mitogen-activated protein kinase |
| MASP-2 | Mannan-binding lectin serine protease 2 |
| MCF | maximum clot firmness |
| MCP-1 | monocyte chemoattractant protein-1 |
| MEA | Multiple Electrode Aggregometry |
| ML | maximum lysis |
| MMP | matrix metalloproteinase |
| MS | mass spectrometry |
| NATEM | non-activated thrombelastometry |
| NOAEL | no observed adverse effect level |
| PAI-1 | plasminogen-activator inhibitor type 1 |
| PAF | platelet activating factor |
| PAK | p21-activated kinase |
| PAP | plasmin-antiplasmin complex |
| PAR | protease activated receptor |
| PC: Act | protein C activity |
| PC: Ag | protein C antigen |
| PCI | protein C inhibitor |
| PDGF | platelet derived growth factor |
| PGE | prostaglandin E |
| PLA(2) | phospholipases A2 |
| PT | prothrombin time |
| RICO | ristocetin cofactor |
| ROTEM | rotation thrombelastography |
| SEM | standard error of mean |
| SDS-PAGE | sodium dodecyl sulfate polyacrylamide gel electrophoresis |
| SF | soluble fibrin |

*List of abbreviations*

| | |
|---|---|
| TAFI | thrombin-activatable fibrinolysis inhibitor |
| TAT | thrombin antithrombin complexes |
| TCT | thrombin clotting time |
| TF | tissue factor |
| TFPI | tissue factor–pathway inhibitor |
| TGFß | tumor growth factor ß |
| TM | thrombomodulin |
| TNF-α | tumor necrosis factor α |
| tPA | tissue plasminogen activator |
| TT | thrombin time |
| UFH | unfractionated heparin |
| VEGF | vascular endothelial growth factor |
| VSMC | vascular smooth muscle cell |
| vWF | von Willebrand Factor |

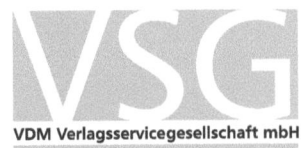

Die VDM Verlagsservicegesellschaft sucht für wissenschaftliche Verlage abgeschlossene und herausragende

## Dissertationen, Habilitationen, Diplomarbeiten, Master Theses, Magisterarbeiten usw.

### für die kostenlose Publikation als Fachbuch.

Sie verfügen über eine Arbeit, die hohen inhaltlichen und formalen Ansprüchen genügt, und haben Interesse an einer honorarvergüteten Publikation?

Dann senden Sie bitte erste Informationen über sich und Ihre Arbeit per Email an *info@vdm-vsg.de*.

**Sie erhalten kurzfristig unser Feedback!**

VDM Verlagsservicegesellschaft mbH
Dudweiler Landstr. 99　　　　　　　Telefon +49 681 3720 174
D - 66123 Saarbrücken　　　　　　　Fax　　　+49 681 3720 1749
**www.vdm-vsg.de**

Die VDM Verlagsservicegesellschaft mbH vertritt

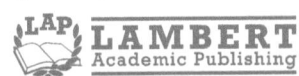
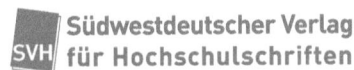

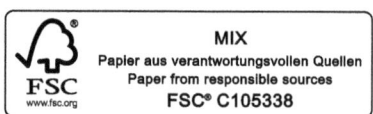

Printed by Books on Demand GmbH, Norderstedt / Germany